THE 1918-1919 PANDEMIC OF INFLUENZA

The Urban Impact in the Western World

THE 1918-1919 PANDEMIC OF INFLUENZA

The Urban Impact in the Western World

Edited by

Fred R. van Hartesveldt

The Edwin Mellen Press
Lewiston/Queenston/Lampeter

Library of Congress Cataloging-in-Publication Data

The 1918-1919 pandemic of influenza : the urban impact in the western world / edited by Fred R. van Hartesveldt.
p. cm.
Includes bibliographical references.
ISBN 0-7734-9195-3
1. Influenza--Epidemiology. I. Van Hartesveldt, Fred R.
RA644.I6A17 1993
614.5'18'09041--dc20

92-35323
CIP

A CIP catalog record for this book
is available from the British Library.

The Edwin Mellen Press
Box 450
Lewiston, New York
USA 14092

The Edwin Mellen Press
Box 67
Queenston, Ontario
CANADA L0S 1L0

Edwin Mellen Press, Ltd.
Lampeter, Dyfed, Wales
UNITED KINGDOM SA48 7DY

Printed in the United States of America

Table of Contents

Acknowledgements

Editors, like authors, generally owe many thank yous. Only a few can be made. Of the few in this case, the contributors to the volume must come first. Particularly for those involved from the beginning, the project has been a long one, but all have been patient and supportive throughout. Richard Peterson, who joined to replace someone who was forced to withdraw, and I owe a particular debt of gratitude. Professor Peterson had written an essay that could easily be revised to fit into this volume, but had submitted it to a journal. The editor, Dr. Doyce B. Nunis, Jr., graciously released the article so that it might appear here.[1]

Personally, I must acknowledge several people. My professor, Robert R. Rea, taught me what I know of being a historian. I should have listened more often. The chairman of my department at Fort Valley State College, Donnie D. Bellamy, supported the project in many ways from beginning to end. My friend, Jerry Page, himself an editor, gave me advice that, when I was smart enough to take it, was invariably good. Finally, my wife, Mary Ann, not only put up with my preoccupation but spent hours proofreading. Greater love hath no woman.

Errors are the responsibility of those of us who wrote and edited, but help avoiding, at least some, was much appreciated.

---

[1]The original version may be seen as "The Spanish Influenza Epidemic in San Diego, 1918-19," *Southern California Quarterly* 71 (Spring, 1989): 89-105.

Chapter 1: Introduction

Fred R. van Hartesveldt

Toward the end of fifty-one months that Wilfred Owen called "carnage incomparable and human squander" and the less sensitive called World War I, influenza began to spread across the world. It was unfairly tagged "Spanish Flu" because the outbreak in Spain was the first to be recognized as serious (the King's case, though not fatal, got much publicity), but it certainly did not originate there.[1] In the midst of the bloodiest war ever known, the early cases were not much noticed. This initially unremarked malady, however, appeared everywhere there were people--even explorers in the polar region suffered. Efforts to determine the numbers killed by pandemics--even those in more recent times--are difficult and never exact.[2] World mortality was estimated at 20,000,000 by Edwin O. Jordan in 1927, and this figure is still often cited.[3] Jordan's estimate, however, is badly flawed, for figures from what is now called the Third World were at best

---

[1]W.I.B. Beveridge, *Influenza: The Last Plague*, rev. ed. (New York, 1978), 40-44. The milder first wave possibly began in the U.S. or China and the more deadly second in Africa or the Near East.

[2]A.S. Monto, "Influenza: Quantifying Morbidity and Mortality," *American Journal of Medicine*, 82 (June 19, 1987): 20-25.

[3]Edwin O. Jordan, *Epidemic Influenza: A Survey* (Chicago, 1927), 214-18. For examples of use of Jordan's figure see Edwin D. Kilbourne, *Influenza* (New York and London, 1987), 14; Kenneth A. White, "Pittsburgh in the Great Epidemic of 1918," *Western Pennsylvania Historical Magazine*, 68 (1985): 221-242.

scanty--Africa may have been left out entirely. His number is certainly very low, and recent studies suggest that it should be doubled.[4] Influenza undoubtedly killed more, in one-fifth the time, than World War I's soldiers managed with all their machine guns, poison gas, and rapid-fire artillery. The chapters that follow all report the inadequacy of previous estimates of morbidity and mortality. The intensive "case-study" approach used here allows such discrepancies to be exposed, although the problems of making estimates combined in many cases with lack of data prevent complete precision in the new figures.

Influenza pandemics frequently come in three waves, and that of 1918-19 did so in many places, striking in summer and winter of 1918 and spring of 1919--although some symptomatic studies suggested that it appeared on the Western Front in 1917 where English doctors labeled it purulent bronchitis.[5] This pattern was not universal, as is noted in several chapters of this volume. In Guatemala City, Rio de Janeiro, and Atlanta, there seems to have been little or no first wave, but as the authors of the chapters about Latin America note, public health services there were so limited that an outbreak of a relatively mild flu, which the first wave generally was, might go unreported. In Marseille the second wave possibly began as early as July, 1918, when in many places the first was not yet over. In Manchester and Frankfurt, however, the three wave pattern was distinct. Although a more consistent pattern would have allowed a more consistent chapter outline, a major goal of this book is to show that supposedly typical patterns tend to break down when examined on the local level.

Although it has been a killer for a very long time--records of pandemics go back to the early 16th century[6]--influenza is not normally

---

[4]K. David Patterson, *Pandemic Influenza, 1700-1900* (Totowa, N.J., 1986), 1; I.D. Mills, "1918-1919 Influenza Pandemic--The Indian Experience," *Indian Economic and Social History Review*, 23 (Jan.-Mar., 1986): 1-40. Mills notes three waves with the second, the worst, killing 17,000,000 in four months.

[5]Kilbourne, 14, 270; P. Fliches, S.L. Baker, W.R. Thompson, "Provisional Notes on the Pathology of the Present Epidemic," *The Lancet*, 2 (Nov. 23, 1918): 697-98.

[6]Kilbourne, 6-7--Table 1.1; F.J. Fisher, "Influenza and Inflation in Tudor England," *Economic History Review*, 18 (Aug., 1965): 120-29.

recognized as a dangerous disease. That the pandemic of 1890-91 killed more people than any other outbreak of disease in the nineteenth century is not even now widely known.[7] The most common symptoms of flu are fever of about 101° F. and a dry cough. About two-thirds of victims have sudden onset with headache and aching muscles in the back and/or legs. Only about one-half of the cases have the sore throat and running nose of the common cold. The typical case lasts three days to a week. The cough and a sense of depression often linger for a week or two after general health is restored.[8] In 1918 all the symptoms tended to be particularly severe, but the high mortality was really a function of complications. Pneumonia was most common, appearing in about 20% of the cases, but bronchitis and other respiratory problems were also often diagnosed. Some investigators sought to attribute a variety of other ills--heart attacks, encephalitis (still regarded as most likely to be associated with flu), and many others to the pandemic, but there is little confirmation, except that miscarriage does seem to have been unusually frequent among pregnant flu sufferers.[9] In 1918, pulmonary lesions and hemorrhages were common, and patients who developed pneumonia tended to have a thick frothy discharge in their lungs which made breathing very difficult. In very severe cases, cyanosis developed and almost always indicated the imminence of death.[10]

The medical profession that faced the pandemic had, over the preceding half century, become quite skilled at diagnosis. The germ theory of disease was firmly established, although the inability to isolate viruses left some room for discussion. Virtually all surgeons had recognized that Joseph

---

[7]Patterson, 72.

[8]Beveridge, 11-13. A popular description of influenza may be found in Stephen S. Hall, "The Flu," *Science 83*, 4 (Nov., 1983): 56-64.

[9]Beveridge, 14.

[10]Medical Research Committee, *Studies of Influenza in Hospitals of the British Armies in France, 1918*. Special Report Series, No. 36 (London, 1919), 11, 49-51; Geoffrey Bourne, "Influenzal Empyema," *Saint Bartholomew's Hospital Journal*, 24 (March, 1919): 62-64; T. H. G. Shore, "The Morbid Anatomy and Pathology of Influenza, based upon 177 Post-Mortem Examinations," *Saint Bartholomew's Hospital Reports*, 54 (1922): 15-16.

Lister's emphasis on antisepsis was the best policy and there was movement toward asepsis in the operating theater. Medicine was on the verge of the breakthroughs that would make it one of the wonders of the modern world. Unfortunately for the ill in 1918, the improvements in treatment had only gotten as far as reducing the likelihood that the physician would harm the patient by his actions. Some drugs like quinine and digitalis had proven valuable. Salvarsan, an arsenic compound, used to treat syphilis since 1910, was the first effective drug specifically for a particular infectious disease. Sadly, not much had been added by 1918: Speaking of a doctor in the 1920s, Lewis Thomas says, "All he had in the bag was a handful of things. Morphine was the most important, the only really indispensable drug in the whole pharmacopoeia."[11]

As is shown in the chapters of this book, doctors tried an enormous variety of treatments for influenza, ranging from bleeding to whiskey to vaccines. Fortunately, bleeding, long a medical standby, was not common by 1918, but it was recommended in French and English medical journals. Most of the other prescriptions were relatively benign. Advocates of vaccines had precedent from successful treatment of other infections, but they commonly ignored Koch's Postulates, established a generation earlier, and based their efforts on Pfieffer's bacillus, which few claimed to be even close to universally present in flu cases. As it had so often in the past, the medical profession escaped its ineptness largely unscathed, although as seen in the chapter about Manchester some embarrassing questions were raised.[12] Doctors were not at fault for much of their ignorance, for no virus would be isolated for more than a decade. Faced by the 1918 epidemic, they were, however, often more concerned for their reputations and fees than for their patients, a situation noted with disgust by Vincent Cronin in his novel *The Citadel* (1937).

---

[11]Lewis Thomas, *The Youngest Science: Notes of a Medicine Watcher* (New York, 1983), 13-15; John P. Dolan and William N. Adams-Smith, *Health and Society: A Documentary History of Medicine* (New York, 1978), 190-93.

[12]Another report of influenza undermining faith in medicine may be found in Nancy Rockafeller, "'In Gauze We Trust': Public Health and Spanish Influenza in the Home Front, Seattle, 1918-1919," *Pacific Northwest Quarterly*, 77 (1986): 104-113.

Cronin's fictional doctor recommended malted milk as a cure for influenza. Real doctors filled the medical journals with claims of cures and paid no attention to what was known of statistical testing. Editors were not more critical of methodology than their contributors. In England, William Farr had introduced some basic statistical analysis in the Registrar General's Office in the mid-19th century. Modern sophistication was in the future, but some tools were at hand and not used. Patients contributed, of course. They expected a prescription, and doctors hoped to ease discomfort and earn a living. They prescribed what they thought would make the ill feel better. Publishing claims of universal cures, however, was going too far.[13] It is hard to read the accounts in this book and not conclude that internal medicine was contributing little support to the population growth of the late 19th and early 20th centuries.

Until the unprecedented virulence of the 1918 virus became clear, most people paid the disease limited attention. The lack of concern was fostered by the fact that the first wave, although most infectious, was less deadly than the subsequent ones, though all had worse morbidity and mortality than previous pandemics. Worse than just the high number of cases--one scholar suggests that perhaps one-half of the human race was infected[14]--and mortality of the 1918-19 outbreak was its tendency to be most deadly among those 20 to 40 years of age. Although there was some tendency in the 1890-91 pandemic for there to be more deaths among younger-adult groups than in the past, those over sixty also suffered unusually badly, with those under twenty being unusually safe.[15] This tendency for mortality to peak at around age 35, as indicated in all the chapters of this volume, was greatly exaggerated in 1918-19. Approximately one-half of the deaths were among the 20 to 40 group, while in England women over 80 had

---

[13]Edward Shorter, *Bedside Manners: The Troubled History of Doctors and Patients* (New York, 1985), 92-98, *passim*; John M. Eyler, *Victorian Social Medicine: The Ideas and Methods of William Farr* (Baltimore and London, 1979), 97-122, *passim*.

[14]Alfred W. Crosby, Jr., "The Pandemic of 1918," in June Osborn (ed.), *Influenza in America, 1918-1976* (New York, 1977), 5.

[15]Kilbourne, 8; F. B. Smith, *The People's Health, 1830-1910* (New York, 1979), 324.

less chance of dying of influenza in 1918 than in 1916.[16] The curious age-specific pattern of mortality certainly added to the impact of the 1918-19 pandemic, for people most needed to meet the emergency and with the most economic potential suffered the worst. This is confirmed by the comments on economic impact in the following chapters.

The aberrant nature of the 1918 virus has never been fully explained. Edwin Jordan, in fact, argued that there was nothing beyond the normal activity of the virus involved. The odd mortality pattern, however, was universal, and the climatic, environmental, and social factors that he thought explained it were not present in all places.[17] The rapid turnover of generations in the organism tends to result in mutations over a relatively short time--it is generally enough different in twenty years to bypass the immune system and cause a new pandemic. Since it was more than a decade after 1918 that the technology for isolating viruses was developed, the strain of that year has never been directly studied, though there have been efforts to obtain it from corpses buried in the permafrost. It was most likely a swine influenza virus "antigenically similar to the . . .virus first isolated by [R. E.] Shope in 1931 . . . .,"[18] though the influenza epizootic among swine in 1918 may represent the transference of the virus from man to animal.

In 1976-77 there was an outbreak of swine flu in the United States which caused much alarm. The government pressed the public, especially those most susceptible to influenza, to get vaccinations even after the vaccine proved unusually dangerous. This was due to the belief, based on antigenic reactions of people who had been exposed in 1918, that the 1976 virus was directly related to the earlier one. Although the outbreak proved short and

---

[16]Beveridge, 30; Registrar General, *Report on the Mortality from Influenza in England and Wales During the Epidemic of 1918-19*. Supplement to the Eighty-First Annual Report of Births, Deaths, and Marriages in England and Wales (London, 1920), 8.

[17]Jordan, 241-44.

[18]Kilbourne, 8.

relatively mild, it was feared that the virulence of 1918 might reappear with similar results.[19]

Historical study of the 1918 pandemic has been spotty. Richard Collier's *The Plague of the Spanish Lady*,[20] is an attempt to study its world-wide impact, but although filled with human interest detail drawn from interviews with people who remember the period, it is essentially anecdotal and quite inadequate. There are technical studies, but these tend to focus on epidemiological and pathological data and/or study the disease over time rather than focusing particularly on 1918.[21] The only country's experiences with the pandemic that have been reasonably covered is the United States. Catherine Anne Porter's novel, *Pale Horse, Pale Rider* (1939) conveys a sense of the tension, fear, and desperation young Americans felt when confronted by the disease. A.A. Hoehling's *The Great Epidemic*[22] is superficial, but Alfred Crosby's *Epidemic and Peace* (recently reissued as *The Forgotten Pandemic*)[23] is an excellent general study of the American experience. Crosby's appropriate focus on the serious problems of San Francisco and Philadelphia, unfortunately, does not give an overall sense of the American urban experience because the focus is on the worst situations. Crosby also suggests a role for the pandemic in the Paris Peace Settlement because U.S. President Woodrow Wilson contracted the disease and suffered from post-recovery depression at a crucial time in the negotiations. In addition to these

---

[19]*Ibid.*, 8, 12; Sally Smith Hughes, *The Virus: A History of the Concept* (London and New York, 1977), 112; George Gray, *The Advancing Front of Medicine* (New York and London, 1941), 178. Extensive discussion of the swine flu situation may be found in Osborn, 29-70 and Richard E. Neustadt and Harvey V. Fineberg, *The Epidemic that Never Was: Policy Making and the Swine Flu Scare* (New York, 1983), *passim*.

[20](New York, 1974).

[21]Kilbourne, *passim*; Beveridge, *passim*.

[22](Boston, 1961).

[23]Alfred W. Crosby, *Epidemic and Peace* (Westport, CT, 1976); *idem.*, *The Forgotten Pandemic* (New York, 1989).

book length studies, there have been a number of articles concerning the pandemic in America.[24]

Beyond the United States much less study of the pandemic has been done. The disease's effects in Africa and New Zealand have also attracted the attention of a number of scholars. Africanists have done much to help prove the original estimates of mortality to be enormous understatements.[25] Historians of Europe and Latin America have not, however, given the pandemic any attention. Other than work contemporaneous or shortly after 1918-19, there is virtually no significant secondary literature about the pandemic's effects on these continents.[26]

It is the intention of this book to pull together some of the pieces of what is known about the pandemic and provide some comparative elements for a more general picture. Outside the United States it is also hoped to provide local studies that would help in the preparation of national and/or regional studies that will eventually allow an understanding of the pandemic as a world event. Considerations of space and finding appropriate contributors resulted in the restriction to the Western World. To ensure the proper expertise for setting the catastrophe in the local socio-economic context, scholars specializing in the history of the countries selected were asked to do studies of influenza in cities. The urban setting was chosen to provide manageable units for study and because concentrations of population are natural foci of infectious disease.

Selection of the cities was largely based on a combination of geographic, economic, and demographic considerations. Most importantly the cities were to stretch across the Western World, starting in Northern Europe and moving across that continent to North America and on through South America. The cities were to be of some significance within their

---

[24]See the bibliography for the listing of these works.

[25]See the bibliography for the listing of these works.

[26]Europeanists have begun to have some comment about the pandemic. See Vincent J. Knapp, *Disease and Its Impact on Modern European History* (Lewiston, N.Y., 1989), 185-89; Martha L. Hildreth, "Contemporary Concepts of Etiology, Therapy, and Prevention in the French Epidemic of 1918-1919," *Social History of Medicine*, 4 (Aug., 1991): 277-94.

countries so that the emergency's effect on the economy and the war, where appropriate, might be measured. It was not considered important that a country's largest city or cities be chosen. In Britain, for instance, the London metropolitan area is broken into a number of small districts which operated nearly independently in health matters. There was too little space available to deal adequately with all the variations. An effort was made, particularly for the United States, to chose cities that had not previously been studied so that original knowledge might be added to what we know of the pandemic.

It was assumed from the beginning that there was no "typical" city. This proved a sound assumption, for experiences on every continent varied. The manifestations and results of the pandemic were much worse in some places--Frankfurt and Manchester--and milder in others--San Diego and Atlanta. The wave pattern was quite distinct in some cities but much less so, to the point of being non-existent, in others. Reactions ranged from much restriction of the public's activities in Manchester to almost none in Lyon to Chicago actually using municipal funds to procure a vaccine for distribution. In Atlanta, city authorities seem to have deliberately understated the seriousness of the situation out of foolish concern for the city's image. These variations show the importance of local studies such as those in this book. While there were some common themes, the situation and response differed from place to place, and before unified national or broader examinations can be done the local differences must be exposed.

To ensure that the book provided readers with some comparative analysis of the pandemic across the enormous geographical area covered, the authors of the essays were asked to include, as far as local resources allowed, some common points. These included a statistical breakdown of morbidity and mortality, with particular attention to the question of a pattern by age. Each essay also contains a description of life during the period of the pandemic and the public health efforts to deal with the problems faced. Finally, each contributor was asked to provide an estimate of the economic impact of the disease on his/her city. By keeping these points in mind, a reader can come away from the volume with a sense of the responses to and effects of the pandemic across the Western World.

Although each chapter contains its author's conclusions, some general results, in addition to the above comments about physicians, may be noted. The oddity of the highest death-rate being at about age thirty-five and the twenty to forty cohort being the worst hit was generally confirmed. Few other patterns emerged with such clarity, for the flu paid little regard to wealth, climate, or other factors. Professors McCreery and Adamo did find a racial pattern. Despite the problem of incomplete data and the long-term mixing of groups, the statistics concerning Rio indicating a significantly increased mortality rate among non-whites--blacks and Indians alike. The problem for Indians is clear in McCreery's work on Guatemala City and was previously noted by Edwin Jordan[27]. Adamo's assertion of a high black mortality supports Jordan's suggestion that American blacks had a much higher mortality rate than whites. The Chicago figures adding a comparison to the mortality of 1917, also indicate that blacks were significantly more likely to die of flu in 1918 than whites. In Atlanta, however, blacks made up about one-third of the population and suffered just about the same proportion of deaths, although as Professor King says, there are reasons to question the exactness of Atlanta's official figures. The more homogeneous populations in the cities of Europe, of course, do not show such patterns.[28]

Evidence of increased Amerindian and black mortality presents some problems. These groups generally had the worst sanitation and least public services of all those studied, which may explain their high death-rates. In Latin America, the mixing of racial groups also makes it difficult to establish a clear pattern. Jordan's data, based in part on insurance records that would surely underrepresent blacks, seem questionable, and the pattern is not confirmed by the records from Atlanta. The rates, especially for Indians, are so high, however, that some genetic propensity for the disease or its complications cannot be ruled out.

---

[27]Jordan, 244-49.

[28]Another study that suggests the lack of patterns is Geoffrey Rice, "Christchurch in the 1918 Influenza Epidemic: A Preliminary Study," *New Zealand Journal of History*, 13 (Oct., 1979): 109-37.

Compared to one another, the performance of public health officials in the cities studied was of mixed quality. Certainly in Manchester and some other cities they provided comfort and nursing to the sick and perhaps reduced infection somewhat by restricting gatherings. The degree of public health activity, however, varied widely among countries--and as the discussions of French cities indicate also within some--and in Latin America was minimal. A key reason for including Guatemala City, which is demographically and economically somewhat different from the other sites, was to offer a contrast in conditions and responses in developed and undeveloped parts of the world. The surprising thing about public health was how little better off the citizens of major modern cities were compared to those where virtually no aid was available. Even in the most developed states, difficulties with unburied bodies and virtual panic were common.

Conclusions concerning the economic impact of the pandemic are difficult. It is clear that contemporary estimates such as the *Daily Mail*'s £120,000,000 for Britain were low perhaps by as much as early mortality estimates.[29] The disruption of services, loss of work-days, and closed establishments were universal.[30] The loss of productivity arising from the more than 20,000,000 deaths just in the Western World is hard even to imagine. The importance of studies like those contained in this book is that by approaching manageable units they provide data that can eventually be combined into more accurate national statistics about just what the pandemic cost. As can be seen from the reports here the amounts are staggering.

Reading the following chapters leaves one with a picture of the Western World almost as helpless before the spread of contagion in the early twentieth century as it had been in the fourteenth when the Black Death marched across it. Although the rate was much lower, the flu killed many more people than its much better known predecessor. In 1918, bodies went unburied--sometimes for weeks--vital services broke down, and people were too frightened to enter the homes of ill relatives even when there was no one

[29] *Daily Mail* (London), Feb. 17, 1919.

[30] For more detail see Fred R. van Hartesveldt, "The Government and the 'Flu': British Public Response to the Epidemic of 1918-1919" *Social Science Perspectives*, I (1986): 46-49.

on his feet to care for the family. There is no comparable situation in the twentieth century, and it is sobering to realize how devastating a disease could be just sixty years ago and how rudimentary the means of dealing with it were. Recent times have given the people of the Developed World a sense of security regarding disease. A.I.D.S. hysteria, however, resulting in infected children being driven from their schools and adults from their jobs has at times seemed an echo of the fearful reactions of 1918. The study of society's reaction to epidemics may then be more than simply academic.

Chapter 2: Frankfurt

Stephen G. Fritz

The latter half of May, 1918, brought unusually cold and rainy weather over much of Western Europe, conditions which mired attacking German troops in the mud of Flanders and threatened to bring their breakthrough in Champagne to a standstill. At the same time, stiff reductions in the weekly bread and meat rations confronted the average German with the all-too-real prospect of starvation, while touching off food strikes and a wave of unrest.[1]

Thus, a regular German newspaper reader might be forgiven if he failed to take much notice of the first reports of a mysterious new disease. This seeming indifference to the onset of the first wave of the worldwide influenza epidemic of 1918-1919 was not unusual. Not until the epidemic was well under way did German authorities themselves realize that the nation was being battered by something extraordinary. This belated recognition resulted from a deficient reporting system, since influenza was not a mandatorily reportable disease (*Meldepflichtig*) for German doctors. Also, many individuals suffering relatively minor cases of the flu did not seek medical assistance. As a consequence, government officials did not know the extent of the disease until it was well under way. Moreover, the demographic effects of the epidemic lay concealed within the larger, unrelenting fury of

---

[1] *Frankfurter Zeitung*, May 4, May 25, 1918; *The Times* (London), May 13, May 17, May 21, June 18, June 20, June 21, June 25, 1918.

the war itself, while the psychological impact was muted by the now grim familiarity of death. The very nature of the disease itself encouraged a certain negligence, since it moved fast, flourished, and disappeared before many people realized the danger. Finally, the enormous disparity between the flu's morbidity and mortality rates tended to produce a false sense of security.[2]

Still, the influenza epidemic produced considerable economic and social difficulties. In seeking to define and clarify these problems, however, the historian is faced with the task of reconstructing and evaluating a past in which the influenza epidemic was considered secondary by contemporaries. In Germany the government suspended publication of many classifications of health and social statistics during the war. In addition, wartime censorship tightened considerably during the course of the war, making even accurate local reporting of negative events problematical.[3] Nonetheless, a reasonable picture of the impact of the influenza epidemic can be pieced together, especially for a specific city, by utilizing newspaper reports, the minutes of city council meetings, letters to city officials, hospital reports, records of medical association meetings, insurance records, and statistical yearbooks published after the war.

Frankfurt am Main in 1918 was a city of considerable significance for the German war effort. With almost half a million people spread along the banks of the Main River, near its juncture with the Rhine, Frankfurt profited from its strategic location and had developed into a key transportation center. Men and war materiel flowed through the city, which also served as the headquarters of a reserve army and the site of numerous military hospitals.[4]

---

[2]Stadtarchiv Frankfurt, Magistratsakte, R1502/3; H. Bogusat, "Die Influenza-Epidemie 1918/19 im Deutschen Reiche," *Arbeiten aus dem Kaiserlich Gesundheitsamt*, 53 (1923): 444, 449; E. Seligmann and G. Wolff, "Die Influenzapandemie in Berlin. Versuch einer statistischen Erfassung," *Zeitschrift für Hygiene und Infektionskrankheiten*, 101 (1923): 157; Alfred W. Crosby, Jr., *Epidemic and Peace* (Westport, CT, 1976), 321.

[3]*Statistisches Jahrbuch für das Deutsche Reich*, Herausgegeben vom Kaiserlichen Statistischen Reichsamte, 38 (1917): V; Bogusat, 444, 449; *New York Times*, June 25, 1918.

[4]*Statistisches Jahrbuch*, 36 (1915): 14.

The Frankfurt region also possessed substantial economic importance. As the headquarters of the Hoechst and Casella concerns, it was one of the foci for the rapidly growing German chemical industry. In addition, the Adam Opel works, one of the key firms affected by the increasing motorization of warfare, was situated in suburban Rüsselsheim. The development of new industries, such as airplanes, and the conversion of existing industrial plants to the manufacture of items such as machine guns, ammunition, artillery pieces, ball bearings, and other such war-related material affected the Frankfurt area. Moreover, Frankfurt still reigned as the traditional center of German banking and finance, although its commercial interests complained bitterly during the war of an increasing shift of financial matters to Berlin. Despite this unwelcome consequence of the war, Frankfurt continued to possess the most important stock exchange in Germany.[5]

The influenza epidemic, however, cared little for economics or finance. Thus, Frankfurt found itself in the path as the flu roared in from the west in the early summer of 1918. Among the general population an air of mystery and apprehension surrounded the disease, which was referred to popularly as *Blitzkatarrh* or the "Spanish sickness." Rumors began to spread of people collapsing unexpectedly of exhaustion and high fever, of abrupt deaths, of the onset of a new plague. Wild accounts surfaced of German soldiers, ill with the flu, being locked in a farm building and pounded to pieces by their own artillery fire. Others asserted that the flu was in reality a vicious new hybrid virus produced by the wartime mixing of high explosives, poisonous gases, filth, and dust. Nor was the popular mood calmed when the menacing disease arrived in Germany accompanied by the most unusual weather in years, snow and frost being reported in the central part of the country, while northern areas suffered four days of torrential rainfall.[6]

---

[5]*Frankfurter Zeitung*, June 19, Oct. 31, Dec. 14, 1918, Jan. 1, Feb. 7, 1919; Leo Grebler and Wilhelm Winkler, *The Cost of the World War to Germany and to Austria-Hungary* (New Haven, 1940), 36-47, 54-69; *The Times* (London), June 25, 1918; *Südeutsche Zeitung*, Jan. 29, 1988.

[6]*Frankfurter Zeitung*, May 24, May 29, May 30, June 1, June 30, July 1, July 3, July 7, 1918; A.A. Hoehling, *The Great Epidemic* (Boston, 1961), 107, 195; *The Times* (London), June 28, 1918.

Surprised by the rapid spread of the flu, the Frankfurt district medical officer (*Bezirkarzt*) released an initial memo on June 30. Designed to calm the local population by giving advice on how to prevent and treat the illness, and by assuring the citizenry that there was no cause for alarm, the circular had little visible impact. Rumors not only persisted, but grew more ominous, as the notion took hold that the disease resulted not from a virus, but from hunger, malnutrition, and exhaustion. German doctors failed to provide reassurance, for they argued among themselves over the origin, nature, and course of the disease.[7]

Amid confusion and uncertainty, the flu assumed epidemic proportions in Frankfurt in the first week of July, when the number of sick skyrocketed. Reports indicated that in some businesses as many as a third to a half of all employees were absent from work. Absences were especially noted among public service employees, armament and munitions workers, and railway and transportation employees. Almost immediately, flu-related production slowdowns and problems in the delivery of raw materials exerted a negative impact economically. Almost as worrisome, moreover, was the explosive spread of the contagion, a development which threatened to overwhelm the ability of the city to cope.[8]

Worse, the medical section of the Frankfurt Food Office (*Lebensmittelamt*) issued an ill-advised statement on July 3. Claiming that clinical observations indicated that the course of this "flu-like" disease was fast and mild, the medical authorities announced that supplements to the food ration would not be made available, nor would additional medical supplies be provided to meet this emergency. Although qualifying its

---

[7]*Frankfurter Zeitung*, June 30, July 1, July 2, July 3, July 7, July 10, July 18, July 20, 1918; *The Times*, (London), July 1, 1918; *New York Times*, June 27, 1918; Bogusat, 449; F. Raffelt, "Ein Rückblick auf die Influenza vom Jahre 1918," *Wiener Klinische Wochenschrift*, 33 (1920): 335; G. Bergmann, "Die spanische Krankheit ist Influenza vera," *Deutsche Medizinische Wochenschrift*, 44, #34 (August 22, 1918): 933; Edwin O. Jordan, *Epidemic Influenza: A Survey* (Chicago, 1927), 10. In the Ruhr industrial area, workers commonly referred to the influenza as the "hunger disease."

[8]Stadarchiv Frankfurt, Magistratsakte R1502/3; *Frankfurter Zeitung*, July 3, 1918; *The Times* (London), July 4, July 5, July 6, July 8, 1918.

statement somewhat by conceding that "special allowance would be made for those with serious complications," the *Lebensmittelamt* touched a raw nerve.[9]

With deaths multiplying daily, with rumors circulating of thousands dying, and with hospitals filling to capacity, any mention of the scarce food supply produced an immediate sense of popular alarm. To most people, the interplay between hunger and the flu seemed clear. Already weakened by years of nutritional deprivation, the average Frankfurt resident subsisted on roughly 1500 calories per day in the summer of 1918, with 2500 calories daily considered normal. In Frankfurt, the average weight loss per person approached 23% of prewar pounds. Moreover, the meat ration had fallen to about one-quarter of peacetime consumption, the average person received only 7 grams of butter or margarine per week and less than two eggs a month, and milk had practically disappeared from the adult diet. In addition, the bread and potato rations had recently been reduced (to 150 grams of bread and 3 pounds of potatoes per person per week), while prospects for the summer fruit and vegetable harvest appeared dismal.[10]

Exhausted from constant toil and progressive malnutrition, and facing a shortage of doctors and medicine, many people regarded the flu as simply another wartime affliction. In order to calm fears that the flu was a hunger disease, the city authorities publicized a report in early July from Berlin which maintained that the number of people affected by the disease had been greatly exaggerated. More to the point, the report also downplayed any notion that the flu reflected in any way on the poor nutritional conditions in Germany. Still, the Berlin authorities conceded that they, too, remained

[9]Statement of the Frankfurt *Lebensmittelamt* in *Frankfurter Zeitung*, July 3, 1918.

[10]M. Rubner, "Der Gesundheitszustand im Allgemeinen," in F. Bumm (ed.), *Deutschlands Gesundheitsverhältnisse unter dem Einfluss des Weltkriegs* (Stuttgart, Berlin, Leipzig, 1928), I: 71-73; *idem*, "Das Ernährungswesen im Allgemeinen," in Bumm, II: 11-22; Untersuchungsausschuss über die Weltkriegsverantwortlichkeit, "Details Regarding Shortage of Foodstuffs," in Ralph H. Lutz (ed.), *The Causes of the German Collapse in 1918*, trans. W.L. Campbell, Hoover War Library Publications, No. 4 (Stanford University, 1934), 180-87; Grebler, 79-83; Gerd Hardach, *The First World War 1914-1918* (Berkeley, 1977), 119; Rolf Wagenführ, *Die Industriewirtschaft. Entwicklungstendenzen der deutschen und internationalen Industrieproduktion 1860 bis 1932* (Berlin, 1933), 22; *Frankfurter Zeitung* May 4, May 30, July 8, July 20, 1918; *The Times* (London), May 21, June 18, June 20, June 25, July 1, July 11, July 30, 1918; *New York Times*, June 21, June 27, July 9, July 14, 1918.

puzzled as to the pathology of the flu, and did not rule out hunger as a contributory factor.[11]

Further evidence of the explosive mix of the flu and hunger issues was furnished at a meeting of the Frankfurt city council on July 9. Debate initially focused on the growing food shortages and increasing prices (problems aggravated by flu-related difficulties in harvesting and transporting produce to market). Attention then turned specifically to the cause of the flu epidemic, with charges that the contagion resulted from poor nutrition and medical care. A city spokesman sought to sidestep the issue by claiming that, because of the lack of a reporting requirement, the exact number of sick could not be determined. While admitting that the flu had reached alarming levels, city authorities nonetheless emphasized that only 911 cases had officially been reported over the previous two weeks. However, since this figure represented only the most seriously ill who had sought treatment at a city facility, various council members remained unmollified. Under persistent questioning, city officials admitted that the actual number of cases was far above the stated level, indicating that medical claims reported by the district health insurance office (*Ortskrankenkasse*) had risen 100% in comparison with the preceding year. Moreover, not only was the insurance office running a huge budget deficit, but city representatives reluctantly acknowledged that they had little idea of how to deal with the crisis should it continue for a few more weeks.[12]

The rather hapless impression given by the Frankfurt city government found reinforcement in two separate medical conferences convened in Berlin over the next two weeks. At the first, called on July 17 by the Federal Health Council (*Reichsgesundheitsrat*) to deal with the burgeoning influenza crisis in Germany, members admitted that little could be done to stop the spread of the disease, owing to its highly contagious nature. Rather ingenuously, the Health Council also recommended that at the first signs of disease, people

---

[11]Report printed in the *Frankfurter Zeitung*, July 7, 1918; *The Times* (London), July 9, July 16, July 23, 1918.

[12]Minutes of the Frankfurt City Council Meeting, printed in the *Frankfurter Zeitung*, July 10, 1918.

should take to bed and call for medical attention.[13] Practical advice, indeed, but suggestions which the average individual could not possibly follow because of the pressure to maintain production at this, a crucial point in the war, and because of the severe shortage of civilian medical personnel. Just a week later, the second medical conference concluded even more glumly that practically nothing could be done to combat the flu, the only hopeful sign being that the epidemic appeared to be going into a natural decline.[14]

These two conferences quite obviously offered little comfort to anxious German citizens, whether in Frankfurt or elsewhere. However, by the time knowledge of their vulnerability began to sink in among both the general populace and city authorities, this first epidemic wave vanished, receding almost as suddenly as it had arrived. Still, despite the fleeting and arbitrary nature of this initial onslaught, some general observations can be made.

First of all, the relationship between the severe food shortage and the flu outbreak loomed large in the popular mind. Despite government and medical reports to the contrary, public concern over a causal link between malnutrition and the flu never abated. This sense of urgency can readily be understood, since by the summer of 1918 not only was there an insufficient quantity of food, but there had been a sharp decline in the quality as well. This resulted partly from the need to adulterate flour with other ingredients to stretch short rations, but it also reflected difficulties in the harvesting, shipping, and storing of food, problems which were aggravated by man-hours lost because of flu-related work absences.[15] When potatoes or vegetables

[13]Minutes of the meeting of the *Reichsgesundheitsrat*, printed in the *Frankfurter Zeitung*, July 18, 1918.

[14]*Frankfurter Zeitung*, July 25, 1918.

[15]Rubner, "Ernährungswesen," 11-22; *idem*, "Gesundheitszustand," 72-73; Waldemar Zimmerman, "Die Veränderung der Einkommens-und Lebensverhältnisse der Deutschen Arbeiter durch den Krieg," in R. Meerwarth, A. Günther, and W. Zimmermann (eds.), *Die Einwirkung des Krieges auf Bevölkerungsbewegung, Einkommen und Lebenshaltung in Deutschland* (Stuttgart, Leipzig, Berlin, 1932), 429-31; Grebler, 79-83; Lutz, 181-85; Hardach, 119; *Vorwärts*, May 17, 1918; W.G. Müller, "The Internal Situation in Germany During September 1918, Being the Fiftieth Month of the War," in Ralph N. Lutz (ed.), *The Fall of the German Empire*, trans. David G. Rempel and Gertrude Rendtorff (Stanford University, 1932),

arrived spoiled because of interruptions in train service caused by the flu, the average German realized immediately a connection between the epidemic and his diet.

Another relationship between the food shortage and the spread of the flu can also be traced. Although city authorities recommended that people not congregate in crowded public places, since personal contact provided the most favorable way by which to spread the flu, this advice proved hard to follow. After all, in order to receive food rations, one had to cram onto a packed streetcar in order to queue to await distribution. Predictably, this contributed to the spread of the flu to a wider audience.[16]

Contemporary medical reports also tended to be gloomy on the connection between malnutrition and influenza. German doctors, as well as neutral Swedish observers, pointed to the food shortage as the main culprit for a general deterioration in the health and fitness of all classes and age-groups in Germany. They further suggested that secondary infections, in many cases the result of a weakened state of health, accounted for a sizeable proportion of flu-related deaths. One study of influenza mortality indicated that 40% of the victims suffered from significant malnutrition, which had weakened their immune systems and left them vulnerable to secondary infections. Other studies suggested that the degree of one's power of resistance (*Widerstandsfähigkeit*), which would be compromised by malnutrition, proved decisive in the course of the influenza. Many local doctors observed that improvement in diet often produced a favorable influence for combating the flu. Finally, other studies generally confirmed that better nourished people, typically those in smaller towns and rural areas, succumbed less to the flu than did their urban, undernourished counterparts.[17]

II: 105-15; *Frankfurter Zeitung*, June 30, July 3, July 7, Aug. 31, Sept. 13, Sept. 18, 1918; *The Times* (London), July 4, July 5, July 8, July 9, Sept. 4, Sept. 10, Sept. 21, 1918.

[16]M. Hahn, "Influenza, Genickstarre, Tetanus, Weilsche Krankheit," in Bumm, I: 334.

[17]Bogusat, 454-56, 464; F. Prein, "Zur Influenzapandemie 1918," *Zeitschrift für Hygiene und Infektionskrankheiten*, 90 (1920): 96-97; Müller, 107; Hahn, 329-40; E. Roesle, "Die Geburts- und Sterblichkeitsverhältnisse," in Bumm, I: 48-59; *idem*, "The Mortality in Germany, 1913-1921," *Journal of the American Statistical Association*, 20 (1925): 163; Bergmann, 933; H.

Ironically, public concern over the connection between malnutrition and the flu reached an apogee during the first wave, despite the fact that the second wave proved much deadlier. In Frankfurt, this likely resulted from a subsequent increase in the ration allotment, as well as from a preoccupation with other pressing matters in the fall of 1918.

In any case, the first epidemic wave, although mild in comparison with what was to come, nonetheless exacted a toll. Just what the precise cost in lives was in Frankfurt is impossible to determine since accurate and complete statistics are unavailable. Still, some idea of the severity of the epidemic can be reached. In just two private hospitals in Frankfurt, and the city operated at least ten other institutions, 53 patients out of a total of 373 admitted between June and August 1918 died of the flu, a mortality rate of just over 14%. If the ten other city hospitals received roughly similar numbers of influenza patients and suffered the same mortality rate, the death toll would have been just under 400 people. Moreover, these figures would not include those who died of the flu without entering a hospital. In addition, other reports indicate that approximately one-third of the population of Frankfurt fell ill with the flu during the summer.[18] These figures obviously are inexact, but they do provide some idea of the extent of the crisis confronting Frankfurt in the summer of 1918.

In fact, the magnitude of the crisis was such that it overwhelmed city authorities, who attempted only a very limited institutional response at best. City officials, during the summer crisis, largely confined themselves to issuing a few public statements urging calm and downplaying any cause for alarm. Ironically, the one decisive measure taken, that of refusing to release more food and medical supplies, itself contributed to the mood of apprehension. Little attempt, however, was made to check the spread of the flu by closing schools, public offices, the theater, or by restricting access to public transportation. Nor did public health authorities issue other than

---

Selter, "Zur Aetiologie der Influenza," *Deutsche Medizinische Wochenschrift*, 44, #34 (August 22, 1918): 932; Jordan, 11, 219; *Frankfurter Zeitung*, July 7, July 10, 1918; *New York Times*, June 27, 1918.

[18]Frankfurt am Main, Ärztlicher Verein, "Sitzung vom 2 September 1918," *Medizinische Klinik*, 14, #39 (Sept. 29, 1918): 975; Stadtarchiv Frankfurt, Magistratsakte R1502/3.

rudimentary instructions for treating or preventing the flu. Finally, little effort was directed at lessening the spread of the epidemic by restricting the flow of soldiers and civilians into and out of severely infected areas. Admittedly, the official documentation for Frankfurt is less than complete, but the impression created from the information which does exist is one of uncertainty, vacillation, and a certain fatalism on the part of city officials in meeting this crisis.[19]

Table 2.1

Influenza Mortality by Age
(per 1000 population)

	All	*0-1*	*2-5*	*6-15*	*16-30*	*31-50*	*50-60*	*61-*
1918	2.13	0.04	0.10	0.14	0.84	0.62	0.19	0.21
1919	0.74	0.08	0.04	0.03	0.20	0.18	0.06	0.14

Source: *Beiträge zur Statiskik der Stadt Frankfurt am Main. N.F. 12. Tabellarische Übersichten betreffend den Zivilstand der Stadt Frankfurt am Main in den Jahren 1911-1920* (Frankfurt/Main, 1922), ccxvii-ccxviii, ccxlii-ccxliii--Table 10. (Mortality rates compiled by author.)

Stung by criticism of its handling of the summer wave, and worried by the mounting public concern over the perilous state of the food supply, the Frankfurt city government responded in the interregnum between waves with a determined effort to put its house in order. In late August 1918, the Food Office announced tougher regulations governing restaurants and inns, while sharply reminding all vegetable and fruit producers in the Frankfurt area that they were under compulsion to register their production with the proper city office. City officials also sought to improve the delivery of food supplies from the surrounding countryside into Frankfurt. In addition, the city government issued new regulations in early September calling for more support for the unemployed, women, the very young, and the poorest sections of the population. Furthermore, the city announced an aggressive new program designed to alleviate the growing housing crisis by forcing landlords

[19]For a sense of the mood in Frankfurt during the summer flu crisis, see the *Frankfurter Zeitung*, for June through August 1918.

to register vacancies and accept new tenants. In mid-September, Frankfurt authorities also took the twin steps of raising the ration for bread and dried potato preparation (used in stretching flour supplies), and giving tacit approval to the securing of food on a "private basis." Finally, the city government stressed that new directives from Berlin emphasized that the fall crops would be quickly harvested and transported to the people, in order to eliminate problems with waste and spoilage.[20]

Because of these energetic actions, Frankfurt food officials were able to raise rations in the early autumn of 1918, the daily caloric intake increasing to 1800 per person. Thus, despite continued grumbling about the quality of the food supply, Frankfurt found itself better prepared to confront the second wave.[21] When the flu reappeared in mid-October, city authorities reacted with more vigor and dispatch.

Although reports of a renewed influenza onslaught circulated throughout late September, not until mid-October did the whirlwind sweep into Frankfurt. From the outset, it was apparent that this wave of flu was much more virulent than the first. As early as October 12, estimates of the number of ill ran to one-tenth of the adult population of Frankfurt, and the flu had only just arrived. Neighboring Wiesbaden was struck so swiftly that schools were ordered closed immediately and postal service sharply reduced. In Frankfurt, too, the second wave initially targeted workers at the Post and Telegraph Offices, where so many employees contracted the flu, and so few replacements remained, that service was immediately curtailed. School officials responded almost as rapidly to the growing menace, announcing on October 16 that instruction would be suspended indefinitely.[22]

Still, the epidemic spiraled in intensity. Just two days after the school closings, the number of flu cases had risen so dramatically that city hospitals

---

[20]*Frankfurter Zeitung*, Aug. 24, Aug. 31, Sept. 2, Sept. 5, Sept. 19, Sept. 22, Sept. 28, 1918; Friedrich Aereboe, *Der Einfluss des Kriegs aus die Landwirtschaftliche Produktion in Deutschland* (Stuttgart, Berlin, Leipzig, 1927), 83.

[21]*Frankfurter Zeitung*, Oct. 1, Oct. 3, Oct. 4, 1918; Rubner, "Gesundheitszustand," 72.

[22]*Frankfurter Zeitung*, Oct. 12, Oct. 15, Oct. 16, 1918; Stadtarchiv Frankfurt, Magistratsakte R1502/3.

reported extraordinary demands being made on them. The city administration reacted by making available a number of branch facilities in order to quarantine flu patients more effectively and limit the spread of the epidemic. In the interest of public health, city officials also ordered wide concessions made with regard to payment of medical fees at city hospitals, thereby encouraging more of the ill to seek treatment. At the same time, the city health commission (*Gesundheitskommission*) urged people to avoid crowded places, to walk instead of using the street cars, to stay in bed if sick, to go to a hospital immediately in the event of a severe illness, to disinfect, wash, and gargle frequently, and to avoid coughing or sneezing on other people. With the experience of the summer fresh in mind, the Frankfurt Food Office also raised the food ration twice over the next two weeks. Finally, city authorities issued a stream of health tips and advice on how to treat and prevent the flu, with the aim of lessening the anxiety of the Frankfurt population.[23]

Over the next few days, as the epidemic peaked, city officials stepped up their public health efforts. The city health commission urged families to make a special effort to care for the ill in their midst, noting that those who could, should receive treatment at home because of the severe overcrowding of hospitals. At the same time, health authorities appealed for more volunteer nurses. Moreover, the health commission now, for the first time, sought to arrive at some determination of the true extent of the epidemic by requiring the local registrar's offices to issue daily reports regarding flu cases in the city of Frankfurt. In addition, city authorities continued the school closings, postponed most court cases, cancelled many plays and concerts, and sought to limit contact between soldiers and civilians.[24]

Once again, as in the summer, data remain imperfect, since statistics only began to arrive after the peak of the fall wave had passed, and even then

---

[23] *Frankfurter Zeitung*, Oct. 18, Oct. 19, Oct 21, Oct. 22, Oct. 25, 1918; Stadtarchiv Frankfurt, Magistratsakte R1502/3.

[24] Stadtarchiv Frankfurt, Magistratsakte R1502/4; Report of the Frankfurt *Gesundheitskommission*, printed in the *Frankfurter Zeitung*, Oct. 19, 1918; *Frankfurter Zeitung*, Oct. 19, Oct. 20, Oct. 21, Oct. 22, Nov. 11, Nov. 12, Nov. 17, Nov. 27, Nov. 30, 1918.

remained inexact because of limitations in the reporting system. Still, the figures available for the last week in October provide an insight into the frightening nature of this new outbreak. Information reaching the Frankfurt *Gesundheitskommission* indicated that during the period October 21-29, a total of 557 flu cases were received at city institutions. The daily average death toll from October 21-25 numbered 20, which then fell to 13 daily between October 26-29, making for roughly 152 deaths during this period. After the peak of the autumn flu wave had passed, therefore, the mortality rate at city facilities still hovered at 27.3%, or almost twice the rate of the previous outbreak. Even granted that the mortality rate would be higher amongst those brought to a hospital, this figure is striking, since the influenza death rate for Germany as a whole in 1918 has been calculated at 2.93% (United States government statistics, published in 1920, put the German death rate, for the period September 1918-June 1919, at 5.9%). Also indicative of the extent of the outbreak was a sharp rise in the number of claims, as reported by the Frankfurt *Ortskrankenkasse*, which had put the insurance office deeply into debt. In terms of comparison with other cities, Frankfurt suffered a higher death rate than London, where the figure for the last week in October had risen to 20, while in Paris the number of deaths, relative to the size of the city, was proportional to Frankfurt.[25]

In terms of age and sex, in Frankfurt, as elsewhere in Germany, the flu noticeably targeted those between 20 and 50 and, in absolute terms, women. Again, statistics for Frankfurt remain imperfect, but tend to confirm studies of other German cities, which found that men and women in their prime were at highest risk from the flu. In Germany, the number of deaths attributable solely to the flu in 1918 was 185,815, of which 114,581, or 61.7%

---

[25]Stadtarchiv Frankfurt, Magistratsakte R1502/4; Bogusat, 450-51 (Table of influenza deaths from statistics collected by the *Reichsgesundheitsamt*: "Deutsches Reich. Influenzaepidemie 1918. Die Zahl der Sterbefälle an Influenza im Deutschen Reiche und in seinen Landesteilen im Jahre 1918, getrennt nach Altersklassen und Geschlecht."); *Statistisches Jahrbuch*, 44 (1924/1925): 15-16; *New York Times*, Feb. 1, 1920; *Frankfurter Zeitung*, Oct. 21, 1918, Feb. 22, 1919; *The Times* (London), Oct. 24, Oct. 25, Oct. 31, 1918.

came from those aged 20 to 50.[26] In Germany, as elsewhere, the influenza virus evidently caused the victim to produce an extraordinarily strong immune reaction, which overwhelmed the body and flooded the lungs with a killing tide of fluids.[27]

Table 2.2

Influenza Deaths by Age

	All	*0-1*	*2-5*	*6-15*	*16-30*	*31-50*	*51-60*	*61-*
1918	885	17	42	57	349	255	79	86
1919	305	34	17	12	83	74	26	59

Source: *Beiträge zur Statistik der Stadt Frankfurt am Main. N.F. 12. Tabellarische Übersichten betreffend den Zivilstand der Stadt Frankfurt am Main in den Jahren 1911-1920* (Frankfurt/Main, 1922), ccxvi-ccxvii, ccxlii-ccxliii--Table 10.

The gender aspects of the flu were also unusual. Available statistics for Frankfurt confirm a broader pattern prevalent throughout Germany: namely, a higher incidence of mortality for women than men. Over 50,000 more women than men died of the flu or its complications in 1918-1919, which meant that 56% of flu deaths were women. In Frankfurt, where statistics are again sketchy, women accounted for a stunning 72% of all flu deaths in the last week of October 1918.[28] However, these figures do not

[26]Bogusat, 450-51; Roesle, 43, 46-61; Hahn, 337-43; Jordan, 219; H. Lubinski, "Statistische Betrachtungen zur Grippepandemie in Breslau 1918-1922," *Centralblatt für Bakteriologie*, I, Orig., 91 (1923/4): 372; Report of Frankfurt *Gesundheitskommission*, in *Frankfurter Zeitung*, Oct. 19, 1918.

[27]Prein, 97; R. Deussing, "Über die Bedeutung sekundärer Infektionen für die Erkrankungen der Lunge und Pleura während der Influenzapandemie 1918," *Medizinische Klinik*, 14, #39 (Sept. 29, 1918): 960-64; Raffelt, 335; Crosby, 221-22.

[28]*Statistisches Jahrbuch*, 44 (1924/25): 44-49; Stadtarchiv Frankfurt, Magistratsakte R1502/4; Bogusat, 450-51; Jordan, 200-03; Roesle, 40-59.

necessarily indicate a greater female susceptibility to the flu, but likely reflect an anomaly produced by the war. Because of the demands of military service on males, and the relentless slaughter at the front, the German population in 1918 simply contained an over-abundance of women, especially in the principal age groups targeted by the flu. This meant that, in absolute terms, more women than men were exposed, and as a result more women died. In fact, as contemporary local studies illustrated, in the 0-18 and the 50-80 age groups, both of which showed a balanced sex ratio, no significant difference in flu deaths by sex appeared.[29] Thus, women likely had no greater susceptibility to the flu than men. The male population of Germany had simply been so diminished by army service and war mortality that a preponderance of women existed, thus artificially skewing the statistics.

In any case, at the end of October, with the second flu wave subsiding rapidly, city health officials began to loosen restrictions somewhat. The prohibition on public meetings and performances, in effect since October 19, was lifted on November 1, although schools still were not reopened until November 15. Very quickly, too, the epidemic receded as front page news. However, this resulted not from a general disappearance of the flu, but from the disruption occasioned by the collapse of the German government. As early as November 9 a Soldiers Council (*Soldatenrat*) took control of the city of Frankfurt. Thereafter, public attention was diverted to questions of the maintenance of order, securing of the food supply, uncertainty over the nature of the revolution, and apprehension about the looming peace settlement.[30]

Despite these understandable preoccupations, the flu continued to exact a toll, with a sharp flare-up in the second half of November and first part of December. Verification of this recrudescence can be seen in the large numbers of black-bordered death notices reappearing in the local press.

---

[29] Bogusat, 450-51; Medizinalrat Dr. Federschmidt, "Nürnbergs Grippeepidemie in statistischer Hinsicht," *Münchener Medizinische Wochenschrift*, #13 (March 28, 1919), 359-60; Roesle, 44-49; Jordan, 200-03.

[30] *Frankfurter Zeitung*, Oct. 29, Oct. 31, Nov. 6, Nov. 8, Nov. 9, Nov. 10, Nov. 11, Nov. 13, Nov. 17, Nov. 19, Nov. 20, Nov. 22, Nov. 23, Dec. 3, Dec. 4, Dec. 8, Dec. 10, 1918.

Also indicative was a report from the Frankfurt Welfare Office stating that the new outbreak had severely depleted emergency health care funds. Moreover, in the less restrictive atmosphere of post-revolutionary Germany, a whole panoply of curatives, aids, mechanical devices, and insurance schemes were newly publicized. Finally, the renewed impact of the flu can be seen in the fact that funerals of flu victims, both in Frankfurt and other cities, were becoming the scenes of demonstrations and disturbances, often resulting in the looting of food shops.[31]

This latter phenomenon almost certainly reflected a "hidden" cost of the influenza epidemic--the toll it exacted on local economies. Even without the flu epidemic there was a frightening decline in German production during the course of the war. Industrial production as a whole dropped sharply from 1913 to 1918, with the 1918 index of industrial output only about two-thirds of the pre-war level. Quite naturally, consumer goods production plummeted even more dramatically. Textile production declined to just 17% of the 1913 figure, as supplies of cotton and wool plunged to 33% of pre-war inventories. Coal production dropped significantly, as did the construction of new housing, while medicine was also in short supply.[32] Nor was the agricultural situation appreciably brighter. Production of cereal crops such as rye, wheat, oats, and barley hung at 82 to 88% of the pre-war figure, but milk, butter, and meat production fell sharply. Moreover, food prices rose sharply during the war. In Frankfurt, meat and potatoes more than doubled in price, wheat flour climbed 76% and rye flour 91%, butter soared 247%, and eggs shot up a staggering 380%.[33]

---

[31]*Frankfurter Zeitung*, Nov. 12, Nov. 30, Dec. 4, Dec. 6, Dec. 8, Dec. 15, Dec. 20, Dec. 21, Dec. 22, Dec. 25, Dec. 27, 1918, Jan. 4, 1919; *The Times* (London), Nov. 2, 1918; *Volksstimme* (Frankfurt), Dec. 9, 1918; Stadtarchiv Frankfurt, Magistratsakte R1502/5-8, 12.

[32] Wagenführ, 21-23; Grebler, 24-72, 103-04; James Angell, *The Recovery of Germany* (New Haven, 1929), 379, 382, 393; Dr. Abel, "Wohnung und Kleidung," in Bumm, II: 125-44; Dr. H. Thoms, "Arzneiversorgung," in Bumm, II: 145-159.

[33]Aereboe, 75-99; Adolf Günther, "Die Folgen des Krieges für Einkommen und Lebenshaltung der mittleren Volksschichtung Deutschlands," in Meerwarth, 200-209; Zimmermann, "Einkommens-und Lebensverhältnisse," 415-74; Rubner, 3-41; *Statistisches Jahrbuch*, 41 (1920): 130-31.

Within these general statistics lies concealed the specific economic impact of the flu upon Frankfurt. What proportion of the spreading economic breakdown can be attributed solely to the flu is impossible to determine, but common sense dictates some conclusions. During the summer, for example, a third to a half of the Frankfurt work force was estimated to have missed work because of the flu.[34] Since the autumn wave was more severe, lost work time was an even greater problem. Indeed, in February 1919 the Frankfurt *Ortskrankenkasse* reported that over two million work days had been lost in 1918 because of illness, a 10% increase over 1917. The situation was further aggravated by malnutrition, which caused illnesses to linger. Moreover, the effects of malnutrition and influenza sharply reduced the energy level and productive ability of the average worker, leading to a steady decline in output.[35]

More importantly for the average person, the flu caused chronic interruptions in train service, which affected deliveries of already scarce food supplies. By October 29, influenza had idled 45,000 railroad employees in Prussian Hesse, of which Frankfurt was the hub, necessitating a reduction in the number and size of trains coming into the city. Further limitations on service were announced the following day, and again on November 5. By November 8, local authorities were warning grimly of the threat to the food supply occasioned by flu-related transportation difficulties and by the spreading political disorder. Some train service was re-established by the 11th, but it did not provide adequate food supplies, for on November 22 the newly-enlarged Workers and Soldiers Council ordered all households in Frankfurt to turn in food reserves above a prescribed minimum level. The next day bread rations were slashed, and by the 28th the food situation was worsening daily, so much so that in mid-December all types of rations were cut drastically. In addition, the increasing isolation of the city contributed to

---

[34]*Frankfurter Zeitung*, July 3, 1918; *The Times* (London), July 5, 1918.

[35]*Frankfurter Zeitung*, Oct. 21, 1918, Feb. 22, 1919; Wagenführ, 22.

the fact that Frankfurt residents suffered food prices amongst the highest in Germany.[36]

Nor was the shortfall only in food. Shortages of coal forced Frankfurt industry to shorten work hours and city authorities to impose restrictions on the consumption of electricity, limitations which were tightened steadily into January 1919. With industry operating fewer and fewer hours a week, unemployment in Frankfurt soared, posing a threat to public order. As increasing numbers of the unemployed grew restless, spontaneous demonstrations erupted, accompanied by denunciations of hoarding and scattered outbreaks of looting, activities which certainly reflected rising social tensions at least indirectly associated with the flu epidemic. That these tensions did not burst out of control resulted from the strenuous efforts on the part of city officials both to maintain order and to assure a more or less equitable flow of scarce food and fuel resources. Still, by January 1919, with some train service interrupted for a week at a time, and with the city receiving only a quarter of its expected coal supply, the breakdown of the transportation system had put the city in a bleak situation.[37]

Adding to the misery in Frankfurt were problems outside the control of city officials. Not only did the flu idle urban workers, but it also incapacitated farm workers, making the harvesting of fall crops problematic. The quality of the potato crop was thus poor, since much of it had been left in the fields too long, and then had not been transported quickly to market. In mid-November, estimates were that hundreds of thousands of pounds of root crops languished in the ground unharvested because of the shortage of farm labor. Moreover, not only did the maintenance of the Allied blockade intensify German misery, but Frankfurt suffered specifically as a result of the occupation of certain agricultural areas which had formerly supplied dairy

---

[36]*Frankfurter Zeitung*, Oct. 29, Oct. 30, Nov. 5, Nov. 8, Nov. 11, Nov. 17, Nov. 19, Nov. 22, Nov. 23, Nov. 28, Dec. 14, Dec. 20, 1918; *Statistisches Jahrbuch*, 41 (1920): 130-31.

[37]*Frankfurter Zeitung*, Nov. 11, Nov. 12, Nov. 13, Nov. 19, Nov. 20, Nov. 22, Nov. 28, Dec. 4, Dec. 6, Dec. 8, Dec. 10, Dec. 14, Dec. 20, Dec. 31, 1918, Jan. 5, Jan. 7, Jan. 8, Jan. 9, Jan. 10, Jan. 15, Jan. 17, Jan. 30. Feb. 2, Feb. 8, Mar. 3, Mar. 24, 1919. It was estimated in January 1919 that the number of men in Frankfurt seeking jobs was roughly ten times the number of jobs available.

products and food to the city. Finally, the economic impact of the flu was made worse by the fact that the 1918 outbreak primarily affected men and women in their prime working age. Thus, in a cruel irony, those most desperately needed economically were most often the ones struck down by the flu.[38]

Within these harsh economic realities, of course, resided elements of human drama, sorrow and poignancy. Consider the case of Ludwid Rothschid, who spent three years in a French prisoner of war camp and another in Swiss internment, only to return home to Frankfurt in July 1918, at the height of the first flu wave, to be claimed as one of the many victims. Lieutenant Max Strauss, who had cheated death for 51 long months at the front, returned to Frankfurt in the hasty demobilization of December 1918, promptly came down with the flu, and died within a few days. Neither Ludwig Weber nor Jean Wiltmeyer got to enjoy life without war, for both young men, teenagers returning from army service, contracted influenza on the march back into Germany and died before reaching the age of 20. Nor were those who died in February and March of 1919 any better off for having survived the first two onslaughts of the flu epidemic.[39]

These cases represented the human side of the influenza epidemic, a personal sorrow now largely forgotten along with the epidemic itself. Because the flu claimed no really prominent figure, because it was subsumed in war and revolution, because the war itself had brutalized attitudes, the influenza epidemic of 1918-1919 was and remained a paradox. Responsible for the deaths of almost half a million Germans, the flu at the time was only grudgingly acknowledged, and then quickly forgotten.[40] Still, the epidemic

---

[38] *Frankfurter Zeitung*, Nov. 5, Nov. 19, Dec. 20, 1918; Aereboe, 32-40; Bogusat, 452-53; Federschmidt, 360; Dr. Schwenkenbecher, "Beobachtungen bei der Influenzaepidemie 1918," *Medizinische Klinik*, 14, #39 (Sept. 29, 1918): 975; Raffelt, 334; Prein, 97.

[39] *Frankfurter Zeitung*, July 17, Dec. 15, Dec. 20, Dec. 21, 1918, Jan. 14, Feb. 10, Feb. 11, Mar. 2, 1919, Mar. 25, Mar. 26, 1919.

[40] In Germany, all flu-related deaths in 1918 and 1919 have been calculated as 429,496. By contrast, the death total for the U.S. has been estimated at 544,000, England at 123,570, and Spain at 140,451. The epidemic death rate per 1000 population was estimated as follows:

did exact a toll, economically, socially, and personally. Perhaps the lesson to be learned is not that people's memories are faulty, but that a society can absorb only so much suffering, and in 1918 the reservoir of misery in Germany was already overflowing.

Germany-5.9; U.S. 4.2; England-3.7; Spain-6.7. See: *Statistisches Jahrbuch*, 44 (1924/25): 44-49, 15-16 (international section); *New York Times* Feb. 1, 1920.

Chapter 3: Lyon and Marseille

Martha L. Hildreth

The historical record of the 1918-1919 influenza epidemic in France often treats it as an episode in the larger drama of the Great War. French society is portrayed as apathetic in its reaction to the epidemic because it was preoccupied by the war and inured to death and suffering after four years of fighting.[1] Yet, while some military, diplomatic, and epidemiological aspects have been studied, the efforts to confront the epidemic with medical and public action remain largely unexamined.

A close look at the course of the epidemic in Marseille and Lyon shows that public reaction was not apathetic. While their efforts may not have been very effective, physicians and the general public moved forcefully to prevent and treat the disease with a wide variety of old and new remedies. Public health action to curtail the epidemic was perhaps less consistently aggressive. While municipal officials in Lyon took extensive measures in their efforts to stop the spread of the epidemic, the Marseille city government was less energetic.

While the influenza epidemic is certainly a chapter in the story of the Great War, it is also a chapter in the history of culture and disease. The war played a role in limiting the scope of action against the epidemic: there were shortages of medicines, hospital beds, physicians, and various sanitation

---

[1] Jean Delumeau and Yeves Lequin, *Les Malheurs des Temps, histoire des Fléaux et des Calamités en France* (Paris, 1987), 419-20.

equipment and chemicals which were thought to be crucial to the public health effort; the attentions of local governments were absorbed by food supply problems, and the national government was concerned that the epidemic not cause undue alarm and thus interfere with the coming armistice. But efforts to meet the epidemic must also be understood in light of other factors which generally describe the relationship of disease and society. Local politics, cultural and medical understanding of epidemics in general, and of the influenza in particular, the general state of public health institutions and legislation all influenced the nature of the medical and public response. The immediate course of the disease itself, which was, in effect, a problem of shorter term in Lyon and Marseille than elsewhere, also determined public response. Finally, the public reaction to the epidemic must be assessed against the long-term state of urban health problems of epidemic nature.

In early twentieth century France public health was still viewed, as it had been since the late eighteenth century, as primarily an urban problem. Thus national policy placed the major responsibility for public health in the hands of municipalities. This concept underlay the 1902 Public Health Law which gave responsibility for sanitary action to the mayors and communal councils. This law also made death statistics the driving force behind municipal public health action. Mayors and city or communal councils were not required to take public action unless the daily death rate should rise above average for that particular city. The 1902 law, along with the 1893 Medical Practice Act (Loi Chevandier), required that physicians report cause of death to municipal officials; physicians generally complied. These acts also required them to report cases of epidemic disease, based upon a list decreed by the National Public Health Committee. Throughout the nation physicians were notoriously and deliberately lax in doing so.[2] For example, statistics available for Marseille show a total of 681 reported cases of influenza in August-October 1918 at a time when there were 1512 deaths

---

[2]For a discussion of this problem see Martha L. Hildreth, *Doctors, Bureaucrats and Public Health in France* (New York, 1987), 198-201.

attributed to the disease.[3] Influenza was not on the "required" list of reportable diseases even though during the epidemic demands were made that it be added. Instead it was added to the "suggested" list. In the absence of reliable morbidity statistics, mortality statistics were the only reliable guide for city action, but they also provided a convenient excuse for not acting. Except in times of crisis or in the face of consistently and dramatically high death rates, the 1902 law did not force municipalities to take action. Nevertheless some municipalities took the initiative on their own to sponsor sanitation projects and build public health institutions.

In 1918 Marseille and Lyon were, respectively, the second and third largest cities in France. Both cities had undergone very rapid population growth in the nineteenth century, Marseille's population having grown nearly three and a half times, and Lyon's somewhat over threefold between 1800 and 1900.[4] In both cases population growth was fueled by industrialization, and in Marseille also by the colonization of North Africa. Both were essentially working class cities, and in the era before the first World War, were still suffering the legacy of the rapid growth of the nineteenth century with crowded living conditions, very poor housing, and a lack of adequate sewage systems and safe drinking water. The result of these conditions were high rates of death due to tuberculosis and infantile diarrhea, and sporadic outbreaks of waterborne bacterial diseases.

Marseille's public health problems were generally more severe than Lyon's as the statistics on tuberculosis and typhoid attest. Since the late 17th century Marseille suffered from severe water shortages, but massive canal projects completed in 1851 and 1906 brought water first from the Durance and then from the Rhône rivers.[5] Although the problem of supply had been at least partially solved, water quality remained a problem. Unlike some

---

[3]Ministère de l'Intérieur, Direction de l'Assistance et de l'hygiène publique. Relevé numerique concemant les maladies atteints de'affections contagieuses 1918. AD Bouches du Rhône, old classification: M7 390.

[4]William Sewell, *Structure and Mobility: The Men and Women of Marseille, 1820-1870* (Cambridge and New York, 1985), 3.

[5]Raoul Busquet, *Histoire de Marseille* (Paris, 1945), 376.

French cities, in Marseille no filtration system was in use. Bacteriological analysis performed in 1917 and 1918 showed that the canal water was significantly contaminated by fecal matter, decaying animal corpses, and general farm runoff.[6]

Marseille was quite proud of its sewer system, a "*tout-à-l'égout*" model which collected both runoff and household waste water and dumped it into the ocean. However, over 10,000 buildings in the city were not connected to the system. In these areas, and in the suburbs, dry tanks prevailed, emptied by the traditional night carters (who were mostly off to war in this era).[7]

For Marseille the source of disease was the sea, or more precisely the commerce and trade, goods and peoples flowing daily into the port.[8] Thus public health institutions in Marseille focused primarily on the age-old problem of quarantine to keep out the great plagues of the orient. The quarantine system was first established under the *Bureau de Santé* in 1643.[9] The necessity of keeping out diseases brought in from the sea was reinforced by the terrible experience of bubonic plague in 1720. In the early twentieth century, the city added a bacteriological laboratory to the port sanitation services. This laboratory began to accumulate data to support the view of some hygienists that most of the city's major epidemic problems had their sources not from trade, but locally in food and water. As of 1918, no action had been taken on this insight.[10]

Lyon had a more dynamic recent public health history. The period of the French Revolution and the Second Empire both marked eras of

---

[6]Dr. Olmer, "L'hygiène dans les principales communes du département des Bouches-du-Rhône, *Marseille médicale*, 56 (Nov. 1, 1919): 756-966.

[7]*Ibid.*

[8]Patrick Mouton, *La Mort est venue de la Mer* (Paris, 1982).

[9]Françoise Hildesheimer, *Le Bureau de la Santé de Marseille sous l'anciene regime* (Marseille, 1980), 5.

[10]Olmer, 775.

aggressive public health action.[11] During the Second Empire a water project brought filtered drinking water to the city, and dike, bridge and sewer projects greatly improved overall sanitation.[12] The effects of water and sewage projects were evident in the statistics on bacterial water-borne diseases such as typhoid and infantile diarrhea. By 1900, Lyon's city hygiene bureau was second only to Paris' in the thoroughness of its services.[13] Lyon also had one of the nation's more extensive urban hospital systems, as well as an extensive outpatient medical assistance for indigents.[14]

At the turn of the century, the tradition of public health activism in Lyon was furthered by two physician-mayors, Antoine Gailleton (1881-1900) and Victor Augagneur (1900-05). During the war, the city was led by Edouard Herriot, mayor from 1905 to 1957 (except during 1940-44). A major national leader, sometime prime minister, and often a cabinet member, Herriot's mayorship of Lyon has been called a principate. In addition to wide popularity and national political power, Herriot had close personal contacts with the city's public health oriented medical elite, and a great personal interest in sanitation and health care services. Given its powerful mayor and commitment to public health action, it was not surprising that Lyon attempted to stop the influenza epidemic with aggressive action.[15]

---

[11] Olivier Faure, "Physicians in Lyon During the Nineteenth Century: an Extraordinary Social Success," *Journal of Social History*, (Summer, 1977): 509-21; Anne La Berge, "Public Health in the Provinces: Lyon," *Public Health in France and the French Public Health Movement, 1815-1848* (Ph.D. Diss., University of Tennessee, 1974), chapter 8.

[12] Charlene Leonard, *Lyon Transformed, Public Works of the Second Empire 1853-1864* (Berkeley, 1961), 87-110.

[13] Paul Strauss, *La Croisade Sanitaire* (Paris, 1902), 313.

[14] Lyon's system of controlling venereal disease, the *Service sanitaire*, was more famous, or infamous, than her water and sewage system. The *Service sanitaire* required the regular medical inspection of prostitutes, and enforced quarantine and treatment for venereal infection. M. Garin, "Du Service sanitaire de Lyon, sa organisation, et ses résultats pratiques," *Lyon médical*, 31 (1898): 37-49, 120-130.

[15] André Latreille, "Le Principat d'Edouard Herriot," in *Histoire de Lyon et du Lyonnais*, compiled by André Latreille (Toulouse, 1975), 363-87.

According to contemporary medical opinion, the influenza epidemic first appeared in France in May of 1918, having been present in Germany and Switzerland as early as late 1917. Public opinion generally accepted the notion that the scourge was another one of the evils emanating from the Germanic east, and transferred to civilian France by way of the western front. It was widely believed in the medical community that the epidemic struck Spain after France.[16] Nevertheless the name "Spanish Influenza" was attached to the disease possibly because of the publicity given to the case of King Alphonse XIII who was struck by a severe but ultimately non-fatal attack in September of 1918 just as the disease was becoming widespread and deadly in France. In France the first outbreaks of the disease, occurring generally in May-June of 1918, were mild; but in the last half of July, or possibly the beginning of August, a new and much more serious strain appeared.[17] At that time officials admitted that fatalities were high, but guided by the well-known model of the 1889-90 epidemic, it was argued that the victims were principally among the weaker sectors of the population, the elderly and young. Somewhat higher mortality in these groups was due, it was felt, to the stresses of war, its deprivations and massive movements of peoples.[18]

The pattern of the epidemic's onset and early course in Marseille and Lyon provides interesting material for the general understanding of the disease's origin and spread. Contemporary opinion, and subsequent histories, have argued that in Europe the disease generally attacked the military first and then spread to civilian populations. However, because the epidemic spread so rapidly it is difficult to prove this contention.[19] In Lyon

---

[16]Pierre Pruvost, "La Grippe," *Journal de Médecine et de Chirurgie pratique à l'usage des médecins praticiens*, [hereafter: *Journal de Médecine pratique*], 5th series, 90 (Jan. 10, 1919):6-9.

[17]*Le Petit Provinçal* (Marseille), Oct. 3, 1918; *La Dépêche de Lyon*, Oct. 5, 1918. Alfred Crosby has placed the origin of the second deadly wave in "the later part of August, 1918." *Epidemic and Peace, 1918* (Westport, CT, 1976), 37. The evidence from Marseille would place it perhaps as early as mid-July.

[18]Pruvost, 11-12.

[19]For a discussion of the pattern of diffusion and the waves of the epidemic see Crosby, 37.

and Marseille it seems that the early, and generally mild, wave of the epidemic in the spring of 1918 struck civilian and military populations at the same time. But the more deadly wave beginning in the mid-summer and early fall may have had its origins in the military population. The problem of tracing the early progress of the disease and its population of origin are complicated by what seems to have been widespread misdiagnosis in the early months of the epidemic.

In Marseille military physicians claimed that the epidemic began locally among German prisoners of war held at Camp Oddo. Of 2,000 total prisoners in the camp, there were 253 cases in May, 97 in June, 45 in July, and 153 in August of 1918. Most of these cases occurred in prisoners newly arrived from the front. Interrogated prisoners reported that as many as half of their regiments were ill with the disease. This early wave of influenza among the prisoners was mild in spite of their debilitated condition and poor care.[20] From May to the middle of July, none of the prisoners died. However, this was possibly not the first impact of the epidemic. Although unremarked by local authorities in Marseille, the city death statistics indicated the disease was making itself felt in the general population in May of 1918 (see Table 3.1). In that month there was an unseasonable number of deaths, 20, attributed to influenza. A telling sign of the epidemic was that nine of these deaths were in the 20-39 age group.[21] It is clear, from both the death statistics and the records of military physicians, that the relatively mild wave of the disease in the spring and early summer was followed by a suddenly more lethal outbreak in late July or early August.[22]

This new wave of influenza struck most thoroughly among the prisoners of war and the military population. The worst cases with the highest fatalities seemed to occur initially among the newly evacuated

---

[20]M. Huek and A. Bourdillon, "La Grippe chez les prisonniers de guerre à Marseille," *Marseille médical*, 55 (Nov. 1, 1918): 883-85.

[21]*Ibid.*; Prof. Boinet, "Traitement des complications broncho-pulmonaires grippales," *Marseille médical*, 55 (Nov. 1, 1918): 856-57.

[22]Dr. Jouve-Balmelle, "Description clinique de la forme grave de l'épidémie actuelle de grippe à prédominance thoracique," *Marseille médical*, 55 (Nov. 1, 1918): 849-50; Boinet, 860.

German soldiers. At first the gravely ill prisoners and soldiers were diagnosed as cases of typhoid and sent to the wards of Dr. Jove-Balmelle at the Hôpital Michel-Levy (the city hospital). Here Dr. Jove-Balmelle began to suspect that triage physicians had erred. Autopsy results seemed to suggest that influenza, not typhoid, was the cause of death. Between July and September 1918 there were 263 deaths attributed to influenza at the hospital; 170 of these were soldiers or sailors and the remainder prisoners of war and foreign workers attached to the military (primarily North Africans from the French colonies).[23] By the end of September, 1800 total cases had been reported among troops stationed in and around Marseille. Altogether, the military hospital reported 837 cases and 305 deaths in 1918, and 350 cases with 110 deaths in 1919.[24]

In the middle of August some startling fatalities unsettled civilian physicians. Physicians at the city hospitals were alarmed by the tragedy of one Marseille family in which five members fell ill at the same time, and three died. These cases, initially diagnosed as typhus, then cholera, were followed closely; doctors finally concluded that both of the initial diagnoses were wrong. Dr. A. Raybaud of the medical school later claimed that several fatalities occurring among civilians at city hospitals in late July and August, attributed to typhus and to various intestinal infections, were probably caused by influenza.[25]

---

[23]*Ibid.*, 856.

[24]E.L. Montel, "L'Histoire de l'Hôpital militaire de Marseille," in Gaston Rambert, *Les privilèges de la Ville de Marseille* (Paris, 1961), 771.

[25]A. Raybaud, "Le Typhus exanthématiques à Marseille, 1916-1919," *Marseille médical*, 57 (Aug. 1920): 751.

Table 3.1

Marseille Influenza Deaths by Month and Age, 1918-1919

Age Groups

	0-1	*1-19*	*20-39*	*40-59*	*60-*	*Total*
1918						
Jan.	1	0	1	1	24	27
Feb.	0	1	1	1	15	18
Mar.	0	1	3	0	5	9
Apr.	0	0	1	1	1	3
May	0	2	9	5	4	20
June	0	0	3	2	2	7
July	0	1	5	2	4	12
Aug.	2	20	59	35	10	126
Sep.	8	76	326	112	15	537
Oct.	9	145	479	117	49	799
Nov.	1	64	200	73	36	374
Dec.	7	33	205	71	37	353
1919						
Jan.	6	22	118	50	33	229
Feb.	5	28	119	52	34	238
Mar.	1	6	57	20	14	98
Apr.	0	6	14	10	12	42
May.	0	1	8	5	2	16
June	0	1	2	1	0	4
July	1	0	5	0	0	6
Aug.	0	1	3	1	1	6
Sep.	0	0	0	0	0	0
Oct.	0	0	1	0	2	3
Nov.	0	1	6	1	4	12
Dec.	3	25	49	21	18	116
Total	44	434	1,674	581	322	3,055
June 1918-May 1919						
Total	39	402	1,593	549	248	2,831

Source: Département des Bouches du Rhône. Conseil départemental d'hygiène. *Compte Rendu des Travaux de Conseil et des Commissions sanitaires*, 2nd series, 16 (1918): 69-80, 17 (1919): 119-30. AD Douches du Rhône, old classification M7/533.

Local Marseille doctors were also alarmed by an isolated but deadly epidemic among civilian war workers at a gunpowder factory in Port Saint-Louis du Rhône. At this small port, located at the mouth of the Rhône 75 kilometers by land or 2-3 hours by boat from Marseille, from the middle of August to September 9, there were 348 cases and 17 deaths. By mid-September the epidemic was beginning to have a marked impact on the city of Marseille. Although, as discussed above, the available morbidity statistics are notably unreliable as a guide to overall morbidity, these reports provide evidence about the pattern of diffusion. Reported morbidity among soldiers and sailors reached its high point in September with 111 cases reported, and fell to 2 reported cases in October. For the civilian population, 53 cases were reported in August, 153 in September, 281 in October, and 199 in November.[26] This suggests that the second fatal wave spread first among the military population including prisoners of war and military workers and then among civilians.

As in Marseille, the disease was present in the Lyon area long before September. Here too, factory workers in the war industries, foreign workers, and prisoners of war were among the earliest vulnerable groups. City death records show evidence of a brief wave of influenza in the spring, but earlier than in Marseille (see Table 3.2). In March of 1918 there was an unseasonable number of deaths, 38, due to influenza. Sixteen of those were in the 40-59 age group although the majority of victims were aged sixty or more. The March outbreak in Lyon occurred before the first significant

---

[26]Archives Départementales des Bouches-du-Rhône [hereafter AD: Bouches-du-Rhône] M7 421; Ministère de l'Intérieur, Direction de l'Assistance et de l'hygiène publique. Relevé numerique concemant les maladies atteints d'affections contagieuses 1918. AD bouches du Rhône, old classification: M7 390.

arrival of American troops in the nation and therefore lends credence to the notion that the disease came into France from the east, if indeed it was the Spanish Influenza. The president of the departmental public health council reported more than a year afterwards that there had also been localized outbreaks in and around Lyon in April and May with a few fatalities.[27]

In June a major epidemic occurred among troops stationed at Vienne, 30 kilometers south of Lyon on the Rhône. Here most cases occurred in the garrison hospital, where 47 of 350 soldiers recovering from war injuries caught the disease. Military doctors said the disease was also widespread among the civilian population in the same area, especially among Spanish war workers. This epidemic was mild, with illness typically lasting four to six days; no fatalities were reported. On July first a military doctor attached to war industries at Roussillon, 20 kilometers south of Vienne, reported a similar epidemic among prisoners of war and Chinese and Indochinese colonial workers.[28] During the middle two weeks of September a severe epidemic hit several towns and villages 25 to 30 kilometers east of Lyon. Nearly all of a group of new draftees in the area were ill and three died. Whole families were said to be sick at the same time and five of eight employees at the Post Office in Cremieu were out sick.[29] As in Marseille early rumors suggested that one of the awful diseases of the past was on its way: bubonic plague, typhus, or cholera.[30]

---

[27]Dr. Mouret, "Rapport sur l'hygiène publique," *Conseil général de Rhône 1919*, pp. 880-81, AD du Rhône.

[28]Dr. Guinet, "Note sur une petite épidémie de Rhino-Pharyngite à forme grippale," *Lyon médical*, 51 (March, 1919): 163-65.

[29]*Le Nouvelliste de Lyon*, Sept. 23, 1918.

[30]*La Dépêche de Lyon*, Sept. 26, 1918.

Table 3.2
Lyon Influenza Deaths by Month and Age, 1918-1919

	Age Groups					
	0-1	*1-19*	*20-39*	*40-59*	*60-*	*Total*
1918						
Jan.	0	0	0	0	1	1
Feb.	0	0	0	0	1	1
Mar.	0	0	1	16	21	38
Apr.	0	0	0	0	3	3
May	0	0	1	4	11	16
June	0	0	0	5	13	18
July	0	1	1	3	14	19
Aug.	1	1	6	10	4	22
Sep.	1	6	19	38	21	85
Oct.	0	94	348	319	195	956
Nov.	0	23	175	151	22	371
Dec.	6	24	107	116	60	313
1919						
Jan.	5	5	48	51	17	126
Feb.	1	5	33	46	12	97
Mar.	1	9	29	21	4	64
Apr.	0	4	3	4	1	12
May.	0	0	2	5	0	7
June	0	0	0	0	0	0
July	0	0	0	0	0	0
Aug.	0	0	0	1	0	1
Sep.	0	0	2	4	4	10
Oct.	0	0	2	3	1	6
Nov.	0	0	0	0	0	0
Dec.	0	1	1	2	3	7
Total	15	173	779	799	408	2,174
June 1918-May 1919						
Total	15	172	771	769	363	2,090

Source: *Bulletin Municipal de la Ville de Lyon*, 22 (1918) and 23 (1919): mensuelle statistiques.

In both cities the second severe wave of the epidemic hit with what seemed like a horrible suddenness in the fall (see Table 3.2). According to fatality reports, Marseille was struck somewhat ahead of Lyon, with 663 deaths in August and September to Lyon's 107. Eighty per cent of the deaths in Marseille in these months were among people aged 20 to 59. In Lyon the comparable percentage was 68. The undeniably high fatality rates in the population groups generally held to be the most disease-resistant began to convince medical authorities and the general population that this influenza epidemic was notably different from that of 1889-90. One doctor described in a desperate voice terrible mortality among the young women in his clientele. "I have lost in these five weeks more young mothers than I saw die in the previous ten years." Among his 45 nurses, 19 were stricken and 5 taken by the disease.[31] October was the most deadly month: 956 deaths in Lyon and 700 in Marseille attributed directly to influenza; in both cities, more than 70% of these deaths were among victims aged 20 to 59.

Overall, in Marseille age group patterns, as reflected in the death statistics, look very like national patterns, with the highest number of fatalities in the 20-39 age group (see Tables 3.3 and 3.4). Lyon, on the other hand, shows nearly equal numbers of deaths in the two middle adult groups.[32] This discrepancy reflects the much higher number of soldiers, foreign workers, and prisoners of war in Marseille.[33]

Marseille's special role in the war and the different timings of the onset of the second wave in the two cities are suggestive in another way. Although it seems as if the first wave struck Lyon perhaps somewhat before Marseille, the second wave reached Marseille first. Marseille was the main channel for foreign workers and soldiers coming into France (1500-4000 a

[31] Dr. Camescasse, "L'Épidémie de Grippe de 1918," *Revue d'Hygiène et de Police Sanitaire*, 41 (1919): 89-90.

[32] Of course it would be much more enlightening if one could verify these patterns by looking at mortality in relation to the demographic profile of the two cities and of the national population. Given the state of French population statistics for the period, and of contemporary conditions, reconstitution of the population into cohorts is nearly impossible. No census was taken between 1911 and 1920. Furthermore the city populations, particularly in Marseille, were in constant flux during the war with large numbers of military and military workers moving in and out weekly. The mortality patterns and the influenza's proclivity for the young adult age groups are striking nonetheless. The mortality statistics are reinforced by many contemporary observers who lamented the high mortality among France's most productive citizens.

[33] "Recapitulation des situations mensuelles des regions," Archives militaire de Vincennes, 5N/225.

week) from the North African colonies.[34] Army records show that among the four major divisions of the military (Army of the Orient, Army of North Africa, Army of Morocco, Army of the Northeast), the epidemic reached its high point of morbidity in the Moroccan and North African troops in September.[35] Could North Africa have been the locus for the development of the second deadly wave?[36] It should also be noted, however, that in addition to workers and soldiers coming and going from North Africa, Marseille also had many Portuguese workers in transit and a large encampment of American soldiers.

Based upon a conservative delimiting of the epidemic from June 1918 through May 1919, Marseille reported 2,831 and Lyon 2,090 deaths attributed to influenza. The total toll for 1918 and 1919 was 3,055 in Marseille and 2,174 in Lyon. It seems likely that deaths due to the epidemic were under-reported in both cities and in the nation in general. In the two cities, deaths due to respiratory illness in two other categories, pneumonia and "other respiratory diseases" show striking increases and unusual age group patterns between June 1918 and May 1919, as compared to the years 1917 and 1920 (see Figures 2.1 and 2.2). National statistics for 1918 show the same anomalies when compared to other years (see Figures 2.3 and 2.4). The cause of death categories for respiratory diseases included tuberculosis, acute bronchitis, chronic bronchitis, and pneumonia, influenza, and the catchall "other respiratory diseases."[37] The unusually high number of deaths attributed to "pneumonia" and "other respiratory diseases" in Lyon and Marseille suggests that the true number of influenza victims for both cities

---

[34]Archives militaire de Vincennes 7N/2003.

[35]Statistique médical de l'Armée métropolitaine, 1914-1919, (Paris, 1922), 299.

[36]Alfred Crosby noted that the epidemic reached its high point in fatalities among civilians in Sierra Leone in September. Crosby, 38.

[37]French doctors recognized a disease they called "abdominal influenza" but while they claimed to have seen this disease in the 1918-1919 epidemic, they generally described it as present as a complication of the respiratory influenza. In my survey of the case studies of the era, "abdominal influenza," is never mentioned as a cause of death. For more information see Martha L. Hildreth, "The Influenza Epidemic of 1918-1919 in France: Contemporary Concepts of Etiology, Therapy and Prevention," *Social History of Medicine*, 4, (Aug., 19991): 277-94.

should include several hundred more victims. Nationally this could add many thousand victims to the final toll. This did not necessarily result from mistaken diagnoses: a high percentage of fatalities were due to secondary infections. No protocol directed doctors how to assess cause of death in such cases.

The lack of guidelines in assessing cause of death was due in part to confusion over etiology. Physicians generally considered the disease to be microbial and contagious. Some physicians accepted the notion that the microbe was a non-filterable virus as established by the experiments of Lebailly and Nicolle, performed in Tunis in September and October of 1918. Physicians who accepted these findings argued that the laboratory findings of bacteria were indications of secondary infections. However, this finding did not shake the belief of many physicians, including members of the Academy of Medicine, that the disease was bacterial in origin. Pfeiffer's bacillus was a popular candidate because it was generally held responsible for the 1889-90 epidemic.[38] Another popular early notion held that the disease was caused by "a reunion of four microbes: staphylococcus, streptococcus, pneumococcus, and Pfeiffer's bacillus."[39] Research in Vienna, widely reported in France, held that streptococcus bacillus was the culprit. Thus there was no general agreement about the existence or nature of primary and secondary infections. Although ideas about etiology were influenced by new findings in medical bacteriology, general notions of transmission are reminiscent of the ideas of earlier eras.

---

[38]B. Roussy, "Nature et modes d'action de l'agent pathogene infectueux de la grippe ou influenza," *Revue d'hygiène et de médecine preventive*, 41 (Feb. 1919): 104-05; "P.G.," "La Grippe à l'Academic de Médicine," *Journal de médecine pratique*, 90, 5th series (Jan. 10, 1919): 46-47; M. de La Vergre, "Chronique médical, Acquisitions étiologiques," *Archives de médecins et de pharmacie militaires*, 74 (Jan. 1921): 125-26.

[39]Dr. Bouffe de Cordebugle, *Le Radical* (Lyon), Oct. 19, 1918.

Table 3.3

Deaths in Marseille and Lyon
Due to Influenza, "Other Respiratory Diseases," and Pneumonia Age Groups
(Other respiratory diseases excluding tuberculosis, pneumonia and bronchitis)

	Age Groups				
	0-19	*20-39*	*40-59*	*60-*	*Total*
		Lyon			
Influenza	187	771	769	363	2,090
"Other Respiratory"	354	397	545	243	1,539
Pneumonia	128	176	319	187	810
		Marseille			
Influenza	441	1,593	549	248	2,831
"Other Respiratory"	797	641	424	768	2,630
Pneumonia	86	354	155	197	792

Sources: for Lyon, *Bulletin Municipal de la Ville de Lyon*, 22 (1918) and 23 (1919): mensuelle statistiques; for Marseille, Départment des bouches du Rhône. Conseil départemental d'hygiène. *Compte Rendu des Travaux de Conseil et des Commissions sanitaires*, 2nd series, 16 (1918): 69-80; 17 (1919): 119-130. AD Bouches du Rhône, old classification M7/533.

Table 3.4

Deaths in France
Due to Influenza, "Other Respiratory Diseases," and Pneumonia Age Groups

	Age Groups				
	0-19	*20-39*	*40-59*	*60-*	*Total*
Influenza	21,148	40,431	18,542	11,344	91,465
"Other Respiratory"	9,733	11,533	9,347	15,285	45,925
Pneumonia	7,716	13,685	9,074	13,026	43,501

Source: Ministère de l'hygiène et de prévoyance sociales, *Statistiques sanitaire de la France*, 35 (1920): 277-305.

Demands for public health action from the general public, the suggestions of physicians, and the plans of municipal authorities also reflected the endurance of miasmatic and zymotic notions. Because influenza was transmitted so rapidly and generally, touching vast geographical areas simultaneously, it gave credence to the notion of "bad air," or "*foyers insalubres*." It was even felt by some physicians that the experiments of Nicolle and Lebailly might indicate that a "vapor" rather than the microbe was the causal agent. Articles in the mainstream medical press hypothesized that some general "vaporous poison" was "infecting the air." Meteorological conditions were cited as ways of understanding the disease's rapid spread.[40]

Miasmatic ideas were also popular among lay authorities. Piles of garbage in the city were held to be a cause of the disease's diffusion.[41] City officials in Marseille and Lyon demanded that to stop the epidemic the cities undertake a general cleanup of "*foyers d'infections*" which had been created by accumulations of filth, decaying matter and infected dust. In Lyon it was claimed that the rue de la Vilette was hit with a high number of victims because its over-flowing privies were creating "*emanations pestilentielles*."[42]

In Marseille there was a widespread attitude that the city's famous filth was contributing to the disease. Commentators claimed that the Place de la Bourse, whose reconstruction had been abandoned at the beginning of the war, had become a "*foyer d'infection*." Located in the center of the business district at the foot of the old port, it was filled with rubble, pits, and uncovered foundations. The area was being used, in effect, as a vast public latrine. Large numbers of people crossed it every day on planks thrown

---

[40]Roussy, 109-10; Dr. Ormes, "La Grippe dans le Var," *La Dépêche de Lyon*, Sept. 4, 1918.

[41]M. Peillhod, "Situation sanitaire de Lyon," *Bulletin municipal de la Ville de Lyon*, 23 (1919), Annexes, 107-10.

[42]Max Aubray, "Un peu de propreté s.v.p.," *Le Petit Provinçal* Oct. 27, 1918; Conseil municipal de Lyon, Seance, Nov. 4, 1918, remarks of M. Sallès, *Bulletin municipal de la Ville de Lyon* 22 annexe, 67.

across the noxious and open holes.[43] Residents of the *quartiers* unconnected to the sewage system assumed that they were being affected more adversely by the epidemic because of the piles of garbage in the streets and overflowing privies.[44] Marseille journalists claimed that the lack of city sanitation engendered poor hygiene habits among the populace, and they held these related conditions to be partially responsible for the epidemic. Journalists remarked that in the poorer districts lacking sewers the residents practiced the "*tout-à-la-rue*," that is, everything being thrown out the windows and into the streets whose cleaners, like the night carters, were off to war. Children, it was claimed, often bypassed the household system by defecating directly in the streets. The notorious habit of Marseille men of spitting on the sidewalks was decried as contributing to the general atmosphere of contagion. The city's own paper money, issued by the Chamber of Commerce to substitute for national currency, which was in short supply, was also criticized as a means of transmission of the epidemic because it was generally in a "greasy and filthy" state. Trash-strewn beaches were also seen as helping to create the "*foyers insalubres*."[45]

Thus in the public mind, the disease was transmitted both by "specific contagion" and by "general contagion," to use the distinctions made by pre-Pasteur medical historians.[46] But the most prevalent theory was one of widespread, pervasive contagion which was simply in the air. Sanitizing the entire atmosphere was a daunting proposition, although one of Marseille's most vocal lay public health activists recommended that the city stop the

---

[43]Olmer, 790.

[44]Conseil général des Bouches du Rhône, Sept. 27, 1918, p. 184: AD Bouches du Rhône, old classification 1 N 269.

[45]"W. A.," "Soyons propres!," *Le Soleil du Midi* (Marseille), Oct. 22, 1918; similar comments were made by Aubray.

[46]For a discussion of this issue see Margaret Pelling, *Cholera, Fever, and English Medicine* (Oxford, 1978), 140-62.

epidemic by outfitting the hoses of the fire department to spray disinfecting mists into the air.[47]

Along with plans to reduce miasmas, public health recommendations were also inspired by the preventive program for tuberculosis. Tuberculosis was the nation's severest disease problem. In Lyon and Marseille, annual deaths from the disease in the years 1917-1920 were not far below the toll of the influenza epidemic in 1918-1919. A national prevention program was begun three decades before the war. The urban program for the poor emphasized outpatient dispensaries which attempted to reform hygiene habits and dispense medications. Both Lyon and Marseille were still in the process of creating these programs when the war broke out, but the ideology of tuberculosis prevention is apparent in the recommendations for preventing influenza, which was, after all, primarily a respiratory disease. This explains the concern in Marseille with spitting on the sidewalks, and in both cities with the problem of contagious dust.

On the 18th of September the Ministry of the Interior sent letters to the prefects warning them that the influenza epidemic was proving to be severe in some cases. The Ministry recommended that physicians be urged to report cases and that departmental health councils be convened to assess the situation locally. Disinfection services, the ministry suggested, should be prepared for an onslaught of cases, and arrangement be made to isolate and care for victims. The local authorities should consider closing large markets, cinemas, theaters, and other meeting places if the situation warranted it.[48] In both Lyon and Marseille, initial action was taken at the end of September.

In Lyon the mayor's office tried to squelch rumors of typhus, cholera, or bubonic plague. The office announced that higher than normal death rates were due to an outbreak of infantile diarrhea due to unseasonable heat, and to a slight epidemic of influenza.[49] At the same time, upon advice of the

[47]Aubray, *Le petit Provinçal*, Oct. 27, 1918.

[48]Département des Bouches du Rhône, Conseil Départemental d'hygiène, Compte rendus des Travaux du Conseil départemental et des Commissions sanitaires, 1918, 2nd series, V. 17: AD Bouches du Rhône, old classification, M7/533, 45-46.

[49]*La Dépêche de Lyon*, Sept. 26, 1918.

City Hygiene Bureau, the mayor's office ordered a number of prohibitions which followed the guidelines issued by the National Public Health Committee. Housewives were told they would be fined for sweeping up dust or beating rugs; damp cleanings were were to be substituted. In addition the Lyonaises were advised to practice measures to disinfect their respiratory tracts and mouths by using gargles, ointments, lozenges and inhalants. People were also told to wash face and hands frequently, not to spit in public, to avoid the cold, fatigue, and over consumption of alcohol. They were also advised to avoid public places where there were dense crowds, noxious or confined air (especially tramways, cafes, railroad cars, theaters and cabarets). In case of illness, they were to call the doctor at first symptoms and to exercise strict hygiene in contacts with victims.[50]

Within a few days of the mayor's decree, it became evident that the epidemic in Lyon was becoming very serious. City services including telephones were greatly disrupted and the number of fatalities was horrifying. Following national directives, the opening of schools was delayed.[51] On October 14, Mayor Herriot took more stringent measures. All funeral processions were forbidden and bodies were to be transported directly to cemeteries (with no more than 24 hour delay); all ceremonies were to be held at graveside. City disinfection services expanded to deal with the epidemic, were to be called in to disinfect sick rooms and bedding. All entertainment and public spectacles were banned; all theaters closed. Public transportation vehicles were to be cleaned with disinfectant every day and their interior air sprayed with disinfectant. Similar procedures were required for all public places from banks and post offices to stores and cafes. Restaurants and cafes were required to disinfect their tables, floors, and sidewalks periodically throughout the day. Finally, the 1917 law on alcoholism was to be rigidly enforced, anyone drunk would be immediately

---

[50]*Lyon Républicain*, Sept. 26, 1918; *Le Nouvelliste de Lyon*, Sept. 26, 1918.

[51]*Lyon Républicain*, Oct. 10, 1918; Dr. Mouret, "L'hygiène publique en 1918," *Conseil général de Rhône* (1919), 879.

arrested, and any cafe or bar where drunkenness was allowed would be immediately closed.[52]

Also on October 14, Herriot ordered the creation of a nursing corps to care for the sick at home. Four city hospitals were admitting military cases for isolation, and two of these, the Croix-Rouge and the Antiqualle were also admitting civilian patients. But beds for civilians were quickly filled. So many people were sick that victims often had no one to care for them. The city called for experienced nurses to apply to the hygiene bureau, offering 10-15 francs per day. The service lasted from October 14 to November 10, and employed 92 nurses. In all 570 families and 2,000 individuals were cared for.[53] The city also obtained supplies of quinine, which were not, however, distributed free of charge, but rather were delivered to pharmacies.[54] In other emergency measures, the city burial service, disinfection service and city hall stayed open extra hours and on Sundays and holidays to register the dead and provide burial for the poor.[55]

Herriot was attacked by the press and by political foes both for taking measures which were deemed to be too stringent and for not doing enough. Herriot defended himself by pointing out that medical authorities were unsure as to the nature of the disease and of its means of transmission; it was, he said, "unfixed" and transmitted by "diffuse agents." Therefore the city was justified in taking measures against all possible means of contagion, insofar as they were able. The majority agreed that a thorough cleanup of the city, advocated by some, was certainly called for, but the city lacked the resources. Herriot complained that the military and national governments refused all requests to free hospital beds for civilians, or to send back horses and carts for emergency street cleaning. He had even requested prisoners of war to

---

[52]*Le Nouvelliste de Lyon*, Oct. 14, 1918; "Decree of Oct. 14," *Bulletin municipal de la Ville de Lyon*, N. 1165 (Oct. 27, 1918); *La Dépêche de Lyon*, Oct. 14, 1918.

[53]"Bureau municipal d'hygiène et de statistique," *Ville de Lyon, Documents municipales* (Lyon, 1921), 9-13; Edouard Herriot, "Approbation des dépenses necessités par l'épidémie de la grippe," *Bulletin municipal de la Ville de Lyon*, 22, No. 1174 (Dec. 20, 1918).

[54]*La Dépêche de Lyon*, Oct. 28, 1918.

[55]*La Nouvelliste de Lyon*, Nov. 3, 1918.

serve in this task but was refused.[56] The personnel of the city sanitation service had been transformed into an anti-aircraft defense squad. They never saw any action, but military authorities refused to release them to their former duties until the war was over.[57]

City disinfection services were quickly overwhelmed, in spite of efforts to increase them. In normal times, the monthly average of disinfections was 137. Between October 1918 and January 1919 the monthly average was 315, and ninety-two per cent of these operations were carried out for influenza or complications. The municipal hygiene bureau, which received requests for disinfections from physicians and families, decided in early October that it would have to turn down requests for influenza cases unless there was a death or a clear case of secondary infection involving pneumonia or bronchial-pneumonia. This decision, in part a response to scarce resources, was also due to a growing recognition that transmission of the primary infection could not be controlled by disinfecting rooms, linens, and clothing.[58]

In Marseille city and departmental authorities were slower to take action even though the epidemic was initially worse than in Lyon. On September 12, a warning was given to the mayor's office by Dr. Astros, a member of the municipal public health council and one of the city's most prominent physicians, as a result of his investigation of the epidemic in Port Saint Louis du Rhône. Mayor Eugène Pierre insisted, however, that no action was necessary in the city since the weekly death statistics were not above average.[59]

---

[56]Edouard Herriot, Conseil municipal, Seance Dec. 23, 1918, *Bulletin Municipal de la Ville de Lyon*, 23 (1919): Annexes, 107-110.

[57]*Ibid.*

[58]Dr. Mouret, "Hygiène publique en 1919," *Conseil général de Rhône*, (1919), 880-82; "Désinefections opérés par le Bureau d'hygiène," (monthly reports) *Bulletin municipal de Lyon*, 22-23 (1918-1919).

[59]Grippe Espangnol, correspondence between the prefect and the Minister of the Interior, Sept., 1918: AD Bouches-du-Rhône M7 421.

On September 26 at a meeting of the departmental council, the prefect, Lucien Saint, also refused to become alarmed, making the same statistical argument to departmental councilors who insisted that some action be taken. The concerned councilors represented cantons outside of the city; they feared that the general filth of Marseille would make it a "*foyer insalubre*," which could harbor the epidemic and spread it to neighboring areas. Their critical view of the city's unsanitary conditions compelled the city's councilors to defend Marseille. Thus rather than insisting on action, they reinforced the prefect's argument that death statistics indicated no significant problem within the city limits.[60]

On September 30, mounting fears and criticisms pushed city and departmental officials to act. The prefect convened the departmental public health council to meet with officials from the city hygiene bureau. Advice on the epidemic was publicized: based on national guidelines, the populace was told to practice personal hygiene and avoid crowds and overexertion. No specific prohibitions were issued. Also, as in Lyon, the school opening date was delayed following recommendations from the National Education Ministry.[61]

On October 10, the mayor's office issued its first public pronouncement and official prohibitions. The Mayor decreed that spitting in public and the beating of rugs were forbidden.[62] The decree urged calm, arguing that rumors of typhus, cholera and plague were groundless. Rather, the decree stated, influenza of the same type affecting all of Europe was striking the city. However, the mayor's office insisted, in Marseille it was most often benign although sometimes accompanied by some awful symptoms. The report admitted that deaths sometimes occurred, "an unusual

---

[60]Conseil général du Bouches-du-Rhône, Sept. 27, 1918: AD Bouches-du-Rhône, 1N 209, 185-86.

[61]Département des Bouches-du-Rhône, Conseil départemental d'Hygiène, Compte rendus des Travaux du Conseil départemental et des commissions sanitaires, 1918, 2nd series, V.XVI: AD Bouches-du-Rhône M7 535, 49-51.

[62]*Le Petit Marseillais, Oct. 10, 1918.*

phenomenon which city public health officials could not explain."[63] On October 22, the prefect, Saint, took more stringent measures ordering the daily antiseptic cleaning of public buildings, cafes, and public conveyances.[64]

During the awful month of October, there was loud public criticism in Marseille of the lack of action taken by the city and departmental governments. Much unfavorable comparison was made to Lyon as well as to Grenoble and Turin where more aggressive efforts were in progress. Dr. Arnaud, president of the city hygiene bureau, made a formal demand that Herriot's prohibitions be enacted in Marseille, but city and department authorities demurred.[65] Journalists cited the lack of initiative on the part of the city as another example of the inability of Marseille to keep up with its more aggressive and modern rival, Lyon.[66] They connected the public health situation in Marseille to the city's general apathy in dealing with social issues. One newspaper commented that the mayor's advice to "keep clean and perfume ourselves with phenol," was inadequate in a city whose people were surrounded with so much filth.[67]

Apologists for the local government in Marseille continued to insist that fatalities were not as high as in Lyon and other cities. They also argued that measures which attempted to generally disinfect the atmosphere or to prevent the gathering of crowds were of no use in stopping the disease because of its virulent pattern of diffusion.[68] The mayor's office consistently sought to take the most optimistic position on the epidemic. Privately, city officials in Marseille remarked that they were fearful that stringent public

---

[63]Le Petit Provinçal *(Marseille), Oct. 10, 1918.*

[64]*Ibid.*, Oct 22, 1918.

[65]Département des Bouches-du-Rhône, Conseil départemental d'Hygiène, Compte rendus des Travaux du Conseil départemental et des commissions sanitaires, 1918, 2nd series, V. XVI: AD Bouches-du-Rhône M7 535, 49-51.

[66]*Le Petit Marseillais*, Oct 22, 1918; *Le Petit Provinçal* (Marseille), Oct. 17, 1918.

[67]*Le Soleil de Midi* (Marseille), Oct. 22, 1918.

[68]*Ibid.*, Oct. 27, 1918; *Le Petit Provinçal* (Marseille), Oct. 17, 1918.

action would scare and panic the population.[69] When fatalities in the middle of October reached a level which belied Pierre's picture of a milder epidemic in Marseille, he argued that these statistics were the result of unusually high death rates in the fall, "when the first bad weather takes many old people." Furthermore, Pierre claimed, the statistics were inflated by the large number of recent immigrants who arrived in the city already in poor health. Critics called upon the city to use its police and courts to enforce the disinfectant measures decreed by the prefect. But the city hall refused to do so on the grounds that disinfectants were in short supply, making it impossible for merchants to comply.[70] Even at the end of October, officials were saying, "it isn't wise to get alarmed because the influenza is most often benign."[71]

Few special arrangements were made to aid victims. Dr. Astros of the municipal health council had urged in September that hospital boats be outfitted to deal with the epidemic, but this was never acted upon. The shortage of hospital beds was especially acute. In peace time, Marseille had one bed for every 1,000 population as compared to Lyon's seven. Marseille hospitals, overcrowded in peace time, were doubly so during the war in spite of extensive measures taken to increase bed space. Beds were put in hallways, in dormitories which normally housed students and staff, and layered 2-3 horizontally in specially constructed frames.[72] During the epidemic civilian cases were isolated at the Hôpital de la Conception and military cases at the Hôpital Michel-Levy (Hôpital militaire). But beds were so lacking that only the most acute civilian cases could be accepted.

As elsewhere in the nation, civilian physicians were also in very short supply. The arrival of Dr. Flaissières forced the city to take action to deal with this problem. A former mayor (1892-1902) and leader of the Socialists,

---

[69]Remarks of Pierre Roux, Conseil Général Bouches-du Rhône, Sept. 27, 1918: AD Bouches-du-Rhône, 1N 168, 183.

[70]Max Aubray, "Ou en Marseille à Marseille l'épidémie de Grippe?" *Le Petit Provinçal* (Marseille), Oct. 24, 1918.

[71]*Le Petit Provinçal* (Marseille), Oct. 28, 1918.

[72]M.A. Vidal-Naquet, "Project de Renovation des Etablissements hôspitalières," *Marseille médical*, 57 (Oct. 1920): 1103-1107.

Flaissières was a senator during the war. He was no friend of Pierre's. Working through journalist friends, Flaissières pressured the municipal council into setting up an emergency medical service to provide physicians' care. Physicians were urged to sign up with the municipal hygiene bureau. Desperate families could request their services through the post offices or public telephones. The city provided the mechanism, but no pay for the physicians, who either worked for free or charged when they could expect payment.

If public health and municipal officials sometimes seemed unable to take initiatives to curtail the epidemic, the same cannot be said of efforts by physicians and the general public to treat the disease. A great variety of medications were prescribed by physicians and utilized on their own initiative by the general public. Generally the favored medications of prescription and self-prescription alike were traditional anti-fever remedies and newer antiseptic substances. In the medical establishment, different views of etiology did not create different regimens. Serums, for example, were used both by physicians who believed they were treating a bacterial or multi-bacterial disease, and by those who saw the influenza as having another cause. In any case, because of limited availability serums were not a common therapy.[73]

The culture as a whole put great faith in disinfecting the body as a way to both prevent the disease and to curtail its effects. Government recommendations and private physicians alike told the population to disinfect the nose by using mentholated vaseline, eucalyptus oil, or gum arabic (acacia) inserted in the nostrils, and to disinfect the mouth and respiratory passages by gargling with hydrogen peroxide, chlorine, or menthol in solution. Dentists advertised their services as part of general preventative hygiene against influenza.[74] Professional disinfectors advertised their

---

[73]Dr. Dubard, "Protéothérapie de la grippe," *Journal de Médecine pratique*, 90, 5th series (July 25, 1919): 239-443; Pruvost, 6-16; Henri Philippon "Bactériothérapie de la grippe par les stocks-vaccins mixtes idoés," *Ibid.*, 44-46.

[74]*Le Soleil* (Marseille), Oct. 18, 1918.

services for homes, apartments, and businesses.[75] Purgatives were also widely recommended by physicians to disinfect the bowels; sometimes it was argued that the disinfective purges were aimed at curtailing the development of "abdominal influenza" as a primary infection, other times they were urged as preventing complications.

The general concept was to make the body orifices impenetrable to disease by creating a sort of antiseptic barrier. Only rarely did a commentator argue that the disease was spread in a way that made such efforts futile.[76] A great variety of heavily advertised, over-the-counter remedies were available for disinfecting the body against influenza, from lozenges and gargles to aromatic cigarettes (to disinfect the respiratory tract).[77] Advertising dressed up traditional purgatives as potent anti-bacterial agents. They were often advertised as remedies for "abdominal influenza." These included "Neutrol," "Goudron Dianoux," "Vrometine (utropine)," and "Anadol." Extravagant descriptions and drawings illustrated the power of the drugs to kill microbes in the intestines.[78]

Popular anti-fever remedies included quinine, camphor oil, eucalyptus oil, aspirin, gum arabic, menthol, caffeine, white wine, and rum. Gum arabic, quinine, camphor, and eucalyptus were also touted as antiseptics by physicians and advertisers alike. Camphor and quinine were also viewed as stimulants to the body's natural restorative powers, as were caffeine and alcohol.[79] Alcohol was also sometimes held to be a disinfectant for the

---

[75]*La Dépêche de Lyon*, Oct. 26, 1918; *Le Petit Provinçal* (Marseille), Oct. 28, 1918.

[76]Comments of Dr. Lucien Dubost, *Journal de Médecine pratique*, 90, 5th series (March 25, 1919): 228-29.

[77]*Le Petit Marseillais*, Oct. 15, 1918; Pierre Borel "Contre la Grippe," *Le Soleil du Midi*, Oct. 27, 1918.

[78]A survey of commercial available remedies was based on the advertisement in the popular daily papers of Marseille and Lyon in the period August 1918-February 1919: *Le Petit Provinçal* (Marseille), *Le Petit Marseillais*, *Le Soleil* (Marseille), *Le Nouvelliste de Lyon*, *Lyon Républicain*, *La Dépêche de Lyon*.

[79]"P.P.," "Traitement de la grippe par les injections de quinine," *Journal de Médicine pratique*, 90, 5th series (Oct. 25, 1919): 783.

digestive tract. It was claimed that Bordeaux wine was the preferred influenza preventative in Paris, while rum was the choice of Provence.[80] One physician-historian of influenza pointed out that the true reason standard remedies such as quinine were used by physicians was not because of any proven disinfectant properties but simply because they had seemed effective in the 1889-90 epidemic and previously.[81]

Efforts to disinfect the body and the atmosphere were severely hampered by shortages of the most popular substances: camphor, chlorine, quinine, hydrogen peroxide, and alcohol, as well as formaldehyde, cresol, and carbolic acid, used to disinfect public places and private dwellings.[82] By the end of October all of these had become nearly impossible to obtain in civilian areas. These shortages were loudly decried, and the government heavily criticized for not doing something more to provide needed remedies and chemicals to civilians. However, in truth these shortages probably had little effect on efforts to curtail transmission. Dr. Vincent of the Academy of Medicine advocated this means in October and the news was widely circulated in both cities at the end of October. There is no evidence that the public ever adopted the mask, although it was utilized by staff in the civilian and military hospitals.[83]

In treatment, stimulants of all sorts were also widely used. Among commercial drugs, restoratives and strengtheners included "Phosoco," which contained protein and calcium phosphate, "Phillules de Gip," and various elixirs containing alcohol. Physicians utilized what they viewed as milder stimulants such as alcohol, quinine, eucalyptus, and caffeine as standard therapy to stimulate the body's defenses. In more serious cases, especially in the presence of heart failure or asphyxia, they injected quinine, camphor,

---

[80]"Une Marseillais," "Chronique parisienne," *Le Petit Provinçal* (Marseille), Nov. 3, 1918.

[81]A.F. Plique, "Le Traitement de la grippe dans les épidémies d'autrefois," *Journal de médicine pratique*, 90, 5th series (Jan. 10, 1919): 36-37.

[82]Max Aubray, "Ou en est à Marseille l'épidémie de Grippe?" *Le Petit Provinçal* (Marseille), Oct. 24, 1918.

[83]Borel, *Le Soleil Du Midi*.

digitalis, electragol (silver suspension), cacodylic (arsenic compound), adrenaline, or strychnine.[84] Although the overwhelming concern was to stimulate, sometimes sodium chloride was used to lower the heart rate.[85] Other standard treatments included expectorants, abundant liquids including teas and alcohol, and misting the air around patients' beds. In hospitals thoracic wraps and ointments were used to aid breathing.[86]

Perhaps the most controversial therapy employed by physicians was recourse to bloodletting. Venesection was used during the epidemic to halt asphyxia in cases of severe pulmonary edema. Dr. Paul Ravaut of the Service de Santé in Marseille urged that it also be employed as a general treatment to prevent the development of pulmonary edema. Ravaut recommended the taking of 500-700 cc. both in critical and general cases. Ravaut claimed significant success with this therapy at the Hôpital Michel-Levy (military hospital) in Marseille.[87] Positive recommendation for preventive venesection appeared in the medical journals popular among general practitioners. According to one well-informed medical commentator, it was widely practiced by Marseille's doctors.[88] Some civilian physicians, including Dr. Pagliano, chief of the Hôpital de la Conception in Marseille, objected to routine bloodletting, advocating it only if there was evidence of severe pulmonary congestion.[89]

---

[84]"P.P.," "Traitement de la grippe par les injections de quinine," *Journal de Medicine pratique*, 90, 5th series (Oct. 25, 1919): 783; Victor Audibert et Y. Pintel, "Forme asthenique de la grippe dite 'Espagnol,'" *Marseille médical*, 55 (Nov. 1, 1918): 870-73; Pruvost, 13-15; Jouve-Balmelle, 849-55; J. Camescasse, "La Grippe simple, Traitement et prophylaxie," *Bulletin général de Thérapeutique médical*, 170 (1918-1919): 219; C. Maurice, "Traitement de complications nerveuses post-grippales," *Lyon médical*, 51 (April, 1919): 187-90.

[85]Anonymous review of the work of Dr. Terrarini, *Lyon médical*, 50 (April, 1919): 211.

[86]Plique, 42-45.

[87]Albert Robin, "La Thérapeutique actuelle de la Grippe," *Bulletin général de thérapeutique*, 170 (1918-1919): 249-50; Boinet, 857-59; M. Sicard, "Discussion dur la grippe," *Ibid.*, 890.

[88]Borel, *Le Soleil du Midi*; *Idem*. "La Grippe: Quelques moyens preventitifs et curatifs," *Ibid.*, Oct. 15, 1918; Dr. Giuli, "La Grippe," *Le Petit Provinçal* (Marseille), Oct. 13, 1918.

[89]Dr. Pagliano, "Formes asphyxique de la Grippe, cynoses grippales," *Marseille médical*, 55 (Nov. 1, 1918): 868-70; see also Pruvost, 14-15.

Aside from medical and commercial therapies traditional popular preventatives and remedies called *"herbes de Saint Jeans,"* abounded in the Marseille-Lyon area. Provence, especially lower Provence, is one of the world's great natural herb gardens. Those used against "grippe" included orange syrup, cinnamon, cherry laurel, lime blossom tea, diocodium syrup, thyme in lavender water, hyssop, rosemary, mint, sage, star thistle, and four color vinegar (consisting of camphor, garlic, and various aromatics). Fennel was used as a calmative and rhubarb and sea bindweed as purgatives. A variety of herbs were used in perfumed infusions released into the air and inhaled in order to "purify" or "disinfect." These included rosemary, thyme, and fennel. Herbal substances were infused in teas, *eau de vie*, and wine.[90] Many of the elements in this folk medicine also were present in remedies of official medicine and in drugs sold in general retail.

Garlic was surely the most famous popular remedy of the South. An ancient remedy and cure-all, it was widely utilized in the influenza epidemic, either to be chewed or rubbed into the skin.[91] Traditionally it was held by physicians to be a stimulant, but during the influenza it was also argued as a disinfectant. Some doctors felt it was effective because of its sulfur content.[92]

In both cities the epidemic started to wane as suddenly as it struck. In November there were less than half as many deaths, and the number of deaths declined steadily thereafter. The military health office reported that a third small wave of the epidemic struck in December of 1919 and lasted to April of 1920. Death statistics in Marseille would tend to support this: 301 deaths due to influenza between December, 1919, through February, 1920, with 49 per cent in the 20-29 and 30-59 age groups. No trace of the supposed last wave is seen in the death statistics for Lyon.

Herriot's severe measures did not remain in place for very long. On November 5, theaters were allowed to reopen and funerals resumed. The

[90]George Cauvin, *La Médecin populaire en provence Thès à la faculté de Médecine et de Pharmacie de Lyon* (Nov. 5, 1930), 41-52; Fernand Benoit *La Provence et le Comtat Venaissin-Arts et Traditions populaires* (Paris, 1975), 214-74.

[91]Cauvin, 41-52.

[92]Dr. Daniel LeClerc, "l'Ail préservatif de la Grippe," *Paris médical*, 28 (1918): 448.

number of daily deaths had fallen dramatically in the last week of October. But more striking to the city council was the fact that information from surrounding villages where there were no theaters, nor crowds, nor public transportation, indicated that morbidity and mortality rates were as high as, or even worse than, in the city.[93] In Marseille on November 11, the municipal government seized on lessening death statistics to declare that the epidemic was in abeyance. The Mayor had the local papers publish these statistics showing that the daily fatality rate (including all deaths) had declined from 108 on November 2 to 40 on November 10.[94] The decline of the epidemic coincided with the great news of the armistice, the abdication of the Kaiser and the development of peace terms. Influenza victims continued to die in November and December. Their plight, however, was eclipsed by the larger drama of a nation counting its dead and families seeking desperately for survivors among returning prisoners, or hearing definitive news of a loved one's demise.

In December of 1918, when Herriot assessed Lyon's anti-epidemic measures, he was proud of the city's accomplishment. Yet the program was probably no more effective than Marseille's in stopping the transmission of the disease. Efforts to meet the epidemic, in treatment and prevention, were extensive, even if they were of dubious effect. The epidemic was widely understood as entailing both general and specific contagion, concepts which predate Pasteur. At the same time, the new ideology of anti-bacterial disinfection influenced efforts to both sanitize the general atmosphere and the immediate body. It was generally felt that cleaning up the city streets might curtail general contagion. But since such efforts required large scale public works projects too long delayed and immediate resources largely unavailable due to the war effort, more faith was put in creating an impenetrable disinfectant shield around the body. In Lyon, nonetheless, under Mayor Herriot, the city did what it could to block transmission through

---

[93] *Le Nouvelliste de Lyon*, Nov. 3, 1918; *La Dépêche de Lyon*, Oct. 14, 1918; Edouard Herriot, Conseil municipal, Seance Dec. 23, 1918, *Bulletin Municipal de la Ville de Lyon*, 23 (1919), Annexes, 107-110.

[94] *Le Petit Marseillais*, Nov. 11, 1918.

measures aimed at both general and specific contagion. The more aggressive response of Lyon as compared to Marseille resulted from its established tradition of public health activism and from the great political power and popularity of its mayor. Herriot could dare to issue prohibitions which might irritate his constituents in the short run without fearing reprisal.

Marseille lacked such a powerful and committed mayor, and it lacked a tradition of public health activism. In addition, Marseille's public health activity was hampered by its old orientation toward quarantine, toward preventing the entry of disease from the sea. Moreover, the influenza's appearance in Marseille, as well as in Lyon, was brief. After its sudden onset in September, it fell off dramatically in November. By January, 1919, fatalities were not far above the usual number of deaths due to respiratory ailments for that season. If the high rates of death had continued longer, one can imagine that authorities in Marseille might have taken more serious action, given the increasing amount of pressure from the press and from people like Dr. Flaissières.

The influenza was also, in a broad sense, a passing episode in the larger picture of urban public health conditions; it was a dramatic but brief event as compared to the continued severe problems of tuberculosis and water-borne bacterial diseases. The cities of Lyon and Marseille soon put both the epidemic and the war behind them. In the 1920s and 1930s public health authorities in both cities built effective anti-tuberculosis campaigns, and in Marseille serious efforts were begun to solve the water-quality problems.

Figure 3.1

Deaths Due to Pneumonia

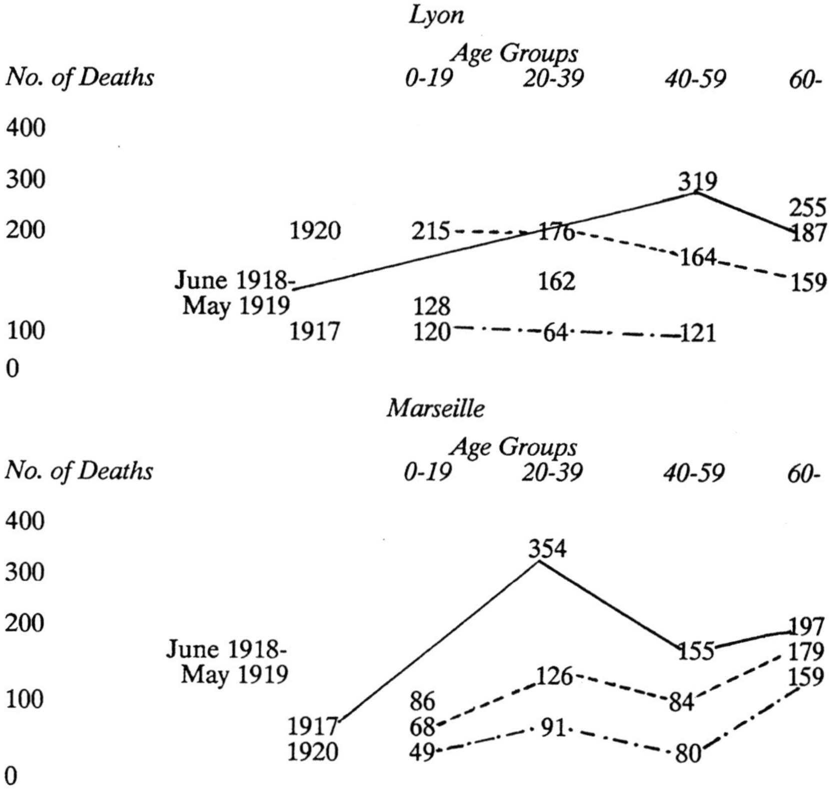

Sources: [see source note for Table III] and Ministère de l'hygiène et de prévoyance sociales, *Statistique sanitaire de la France,* V. 32 (1917) pp. 29-34, V. 35 (1920) pp. 69-72.

Figure 3.2

Deaths Due to "Other Respiratory Diseases"
(not including bronchitis, pneumonia, or tuberculosis)

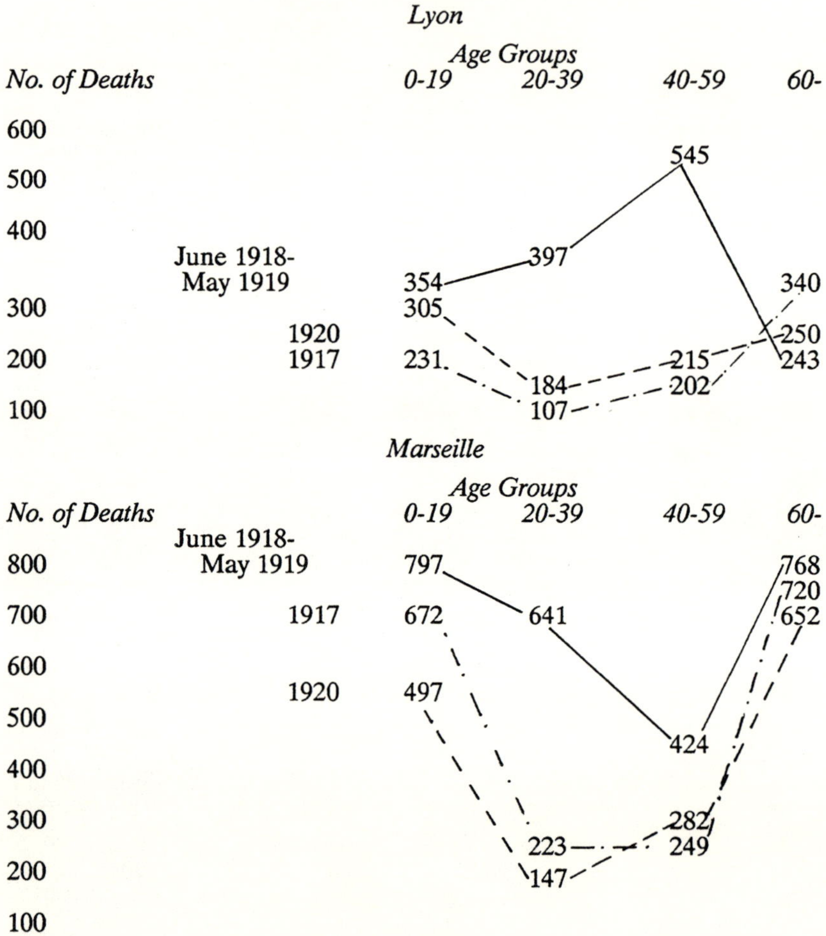

Sources: [see source note for Table III] and Ministère de l'hygiène et de prévoyance sociales, *Statistique sanitaire de la France,* V. 32 (1917) pp. 29-34, V. 35 (1920) pp. 69-72.

Figure 3.3

Deaths Due to Pneumonia in all of France:
1918 Compared to the Average for 1914-1917

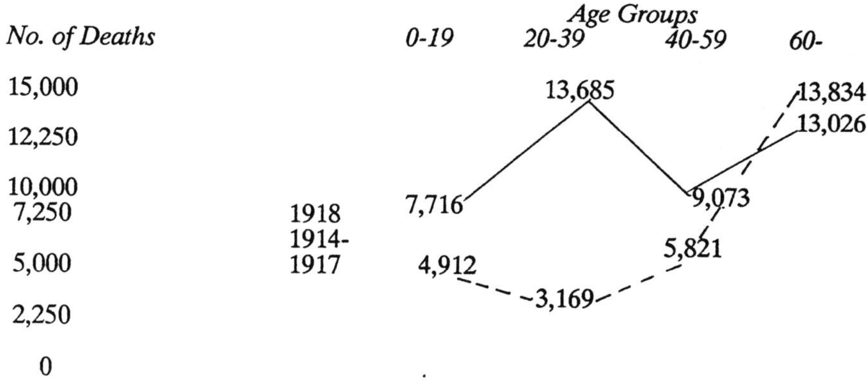

Figure 3.4

Deaths Due to "Other Respiratory Diseases" in all of France:
1918 Compared to the Average for 1914-1917

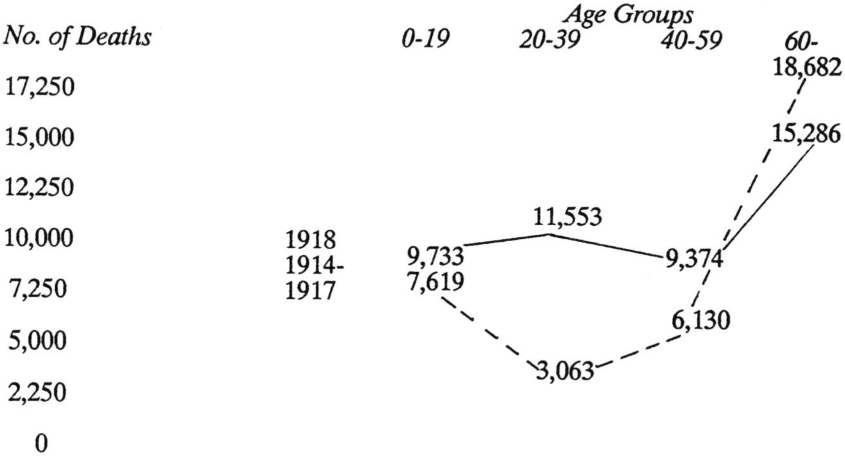

Sources: Ministère de l'hygiène et de prévoyance sociales, *Statistique sanitaire de la France*, V. 35 (1920) pp. 277-305.

Chapter 4: Paris

Diane A. V. Puklin

Observers of the influenza epidemic that appeared in Paris in early fall, 1918, cited the summer's exceptional heat as the premonitory sign of this "Greatest pandemic of influenza the world has ever experienced."[1]

It was agreed that an early, milder variety of the influenza appeared among French troops in April, 1918, presumably transmitted by the American Expeditionary Forces stationed near Bordeaux.[2] Taking immediate precautions, the *Service de Santé-Militaire* called for reports of all cases.[3]

Traveling home that hot July, French soldiers transmitted a more serious strain of the grippe, as it was commonly called in France. July statistics for Paris registered 52 deaths from grippe, a sharp climb from the 19 case average for influenza for that month.[4] Later reports of rising numbers of grippe mortality coincided with the return of Parisiens from their

---

[1]Charles H. Stuart-Harris, Geoffrey C. Schild, John S. Oxford, *Influenza, The Viruses and the Disease*, 2nd ed. (Baltimore, 1985), 119; Pierre Lereboullet, *La Grippe, Clinique, Prophylaxie, Traitement* (Paris, 1926), 11.

[2]Alfred W. Crosby, Jr., *Epidemic and Peace, 1918* (Westport, CT, 1976), 25; Stuart-Harris, *et al.*, 119.

[3]Crosby, 25.

[4]Louis Cruveilheir, "La Grippe à Paris en 1918, Statistique, Bacteriologie, Hygiène," *Le Journal Médical Français*, 8 (1919): 27.

August vacations.[5] By mid-September, the mortality rate was rising exponentially. A directive from the Minister of the Interior warned of the disease's potential threat and urged physicians to recognize the *declaration obligatoire* to report all cases. The directive defined measures to halt the disease's spread and advised restrictions of public gatherings.[6]

The last week of September registered 192 deaths from the grippe. Parisiens numbering 3,734 died from the grippe between October 5 and November 2; this was five times the average for this period. Total deaths from pulmonary disease were seven times above the seasonal average.[7] Then, as precipitiously as the numbers had risen, by mid-November, they fell. More fortunate than other parts of France, Paris enjoyed a significantly lower incidence of grippe mortality in December: 168 deaths from grippe and 133 from pulmonary disease. Both figures were below the norm for that month.[8] All told, Paris reported 7,777 deaths from the grippe in 1918 and 2,722 in 1919--despite the brief resurgence of the disease in late January.[9] Subsequent to its January, 1919, reappearance, grippe was reported in scattered clusters during the winter of 1923-24 and again during the winter of 1924-25. None of these reappearances reached the morbidity, mortality, or severity of the original fall, 1918, episode.

---

[5]Lereboullet, 12.

[6]France, "Circulaire du Ministre de l'Intérieur aux Préfets, en date du 18 Septembre 1918, au Sujet de la Grippe, "*La Presse Médicale*, 26 (1918): 127-28.

[7]Cruveilheir, 27.

[8]*Ibid.*

[9]Demographie. "Causes de décès par âge et par sexe, 1918, 1919," *Institut National de'Études Démographique*, Paris.

Table 4.1

Influenza Deaths by Age in Paris

	Total	0-1	1-9	10-19	20-29	30-39	40-49	50-59	60-69	70-79	80
1900	592	19	33	14	37	35	45	75	105	139	87
1917	127	4	5	1	6	7	8	30	22	24	15
1918	6394	81	334	767	1882	1664	694	548	314	219	30
1919	2270	46	103	271	512	496	284	279	209	135	27
1920	689	14	30	46	140	187	85	81	56	51	32
1921	145	4	7	14	39	16	20	22	10	10	3

Source: *Annuaire statistique de la ville de Paris.* (Paris, 1902, 1921, 1922, 1925).

Grippe victims usually succumbed to secondary pulmonary complications. These unfortunate individuals represented close to 10% of all those who contracted the influenza and half of those who developed complications. In the other 90% of cases, grippe acted much like common influenza.[10]

With France's civilian supply of physicians drained by the war, the majority of grippe patients received treatment within their households, their cases remaining unreported. That grippe was sometimes misdiagnosed as cholera further compromised an assessment of its morbidity;[11] this confusion occurred early in the epidemic when the gastrointestinal involvement remained largely unrecognized. Physicians also confused grippe with dysentery, which had reached epidemic proportions in Paris in October.[12] Finally, physicians' opposition to reporting contagious disease rendered any morbidity count totally unreliable. More on this complication later.

---

[10]W.I.B. Beveridge, *Influenza: The Last Great Plague* (New York, 1977), 14-15; Lereboullet, 99.

[11]Francis Heckel, "Nouvelles Observations sur la Grippe Actuelle," *L'Illustration*, 151 (Nov. 9, 1918), 449.

[12]*Figaro*, Oct. 11, 1918; Beveridge, 14-15; R. Wurtz et F. Bezançon, "Note sur l'Épidemie Parisienne de Grippe et sur les Erreurs de Diagnostic, que Certaines Formes Peuvent Entrainer," *Bulletin de l'Académie de Médecine*, 39 (1918): 286-90.

No illusions of immunity could be construed for grippe; unlike cholera and other epidemics that preferred the poor, grippe was nondiscriminatory. Royalty, statesmen, and war heroes occupied places in its mortality statistics as did bourgeoise who practiced the prescribed prophylactic measures; also included were those on the lower end of the socioeconomic spectrum whose numbers usually swelled the ranks of epidemic victims. Nor was age a shield. Grippe had a frightening proclivity for persons in the prime of life--between the ages of 20 and 40; most had been in good health prior to the disease's onset. Their horrible deaths from severe pulmonary complications, particularly those deaths marked by cyanosis due to pulmonary edema, rendered this disease one of the most frightening to visit Paris in decades.

In Paris, the popular media assured public awareness of the epidemic. Repeated reports provided abundant information. Indeed, the enormity of the epidemic was conveyed in reports of mortality statistics and public health measures, advertisements on prophylactic medications, and discussions of medical research on the grippe's cause and treatment. A controlled, objective focus characterized the reporting of the conservative newspaper *Figaro* and the popular, coffee-table magazine, *L'Illustration.*

A lighter tone could be found in the *Mercure de France.* In its pages, historical vignettes on grippe joined names of important persons bedded by the disease, such as Lloyd George and the King of Spain. *Mercure* readers were also informed about home remedies. The onion cure, esthetically suspect but reputedly sound therapeutically, received considerable attention, as did its advocate, Mrs. Hetty Green, "known in New York as America [sic] richest business woman."[13] Mrs. Green claimed that she ate onions daily and never left home without a few in her pocket; she was reported to be in excellent health.

Sensationalism characterized the message of over-the-counter drug advertisements. Seizing an outstanding marketing opportunity, the ads offered simple explanations of the grippe and bold claims of cure. In October, it was reported that Paris pharmacies did a brisk trade in drugs

---

[13]*Mercure de France*, 129 (Sept.-Oct., 1918): 190 (italics *Mercure de France*).

purported to prevent and/or cure the grippe.[14] The Academy of Medicine censured this market play upon the public's concern.[15]

Well-informed about the grippe, Parisiens could still take comfort in the knowledge that the disease presented like benign common influenza in 90% of the cases. Like those on the front lines, they were forced to play the odds. The war presented the most immediate danger. Mirroring this overriding concern, reports from the front dominated the daily press. As Paris's grippe mortality statistics surged, the news from the front brought welcomed signs of peace and the promise of Versailles. The restrained jubilance of this long-awaited turn of events coupled with the generally benign nature of the grippe muted public reaction to this epidemic. Relative to the war coverage, that of the grippe appeared understated. *Figaro* reported on the epidemic when it was a topic at the weekly Academy of Medicine meetings; a synopsis of these meetings appeared on the second page of the newspaper and occupied a portion of a column in this five-column newspaper.

L'Illustration devoted three and one-half pages over a three week period that coincided with the height of the epidemic. Written by Dr. Francis Heckel, this series informed readers on the history, cause, prophylactic measures, and treatments of the disease. The positive message of this series was that prophylactic measures provided good resistance to the infection; even if begun late when the grippe was actually contracted, such measures would at least insure against developing the dreaded secondary complications. Dr. Heckel's message, like that from the front, was upbeat and reassuring. For a war-torn people, the promise of Versailles provided more welcomed news than the grim reports of an epidemic with its mortality statistics; figures of death had been stalking Paris news since 1914. Indeed, in the public mind, which believed the epidemic exposed the war's deleterious impact upon the people's health, the war could also claim the

---

[14]Louise Deletang, *Journal d'une Ouvriere Parisienne pendant la Guerre* (Paris, 1935), 442.

[15]René Dage, "Procès-Verbal de la Réunion de la Commission Nommée pour L'Étude de la Repression de la Publicité Trompeuse," *Revue d'Hygiène et de Police Sanitaire*, 49 (1919): 762-66.

victims of grippe.[16] The constant psychological stress and physical deprivations imposed by the war explained the disease's timely appearance. Some even suspected that the grippe was communicated to France by Germans on the front lines.[17]

Mindful of the public mood, the Paris government deflected public attention from the epidemic. They refrained from imposing restrictions that would either focus public attention on the epidemic's potential dangers or would create inconveniences to further stress the public psyche.[18] Thus measures to control crowds, such as closing theaters, movie houses, and the markets were not implemented. Even sales of items that could be considered harbingers of contagion, such as used linens and bedding, remained unforbidden.[19] Public transportation, strongly implicated in the spread of this contagious disease, continued full operations. Departing briefly from this policy, Paris public schools were dismissed from 26 October to 4 November. This measure received the disapproval of the medical community, which claimed it was enacted too late to be effective.[20]

What the Paris government did not restrict, the Parisiens did not voluntarily avoid. In October, as the epidemic raged, Paris night-life was thriving. The Opera, the Comedie-française, the Opera Comique, the Casino, along with other theaters and popular gatherings, suffered no economic ill effects from the grippe. Meanwhile, legislation favoring the 8-hour day brought crowds of demonstrators together to shout, cough, and otherwise share their outrage and germs. In the brief period that this laissez-faire policy persisted, Paris officials watched the grippe figures peak and then

---

[16]Dr. Leuret, "La Grippe à Bordeaux," *Le Journal Médical Français*, 8 (1919): 21-26; Deletang, 454, 458.

[17]Lereboullet, 12.

[18]Cruveilheir, 31; *Ministre de l'Intérieur*, 128.

[19]Dr. Lassabate, "Lettre," *Revue de'Hygiène et de Police Sanitaire*, 49 (1919): 1202-03.

[20]L. Fortineau, "Quelques Remarques sur la Grippe de 1918-19," *Annales d'Hygiène Publique et de Médicine Legale*, 36 (1921): 69.

drop. By November 11, when the jubilant crowds swarmed into the streets of Paris to celebrate the peace, the epidemic had receded from public concern.

Behind the controlled reactions of the press and government, Paris hospitals attempted to accommodate surging admissions of grippe patients. The infectious nature of the disease compounded the stress on hospital facilities. Provisions had to be implemented to isolate grippe patients and, within the community of grippe patients, to isolate those with pulmonary complications.

On September 25, M. Mesureur, Director of Public Assistance, Paris, communicated the order of the Prefect of Police for the Seine to the Paris hospitals: the hospitals were to set aside beds for grippe patients.[21] Five hospitals responded and together provided a total of 864 beds; 26% of these were stretchers placed in hospital hallways.[22] Isolation wards were quickly constructed, some from plywood, others from canvas and sheet. Compromising these precautions, the government issued only advisements concerning hospital visitors; restrictions were avoided for fear of alarming the public.[23] Critics placed responsibility for the hospital mortality rate--20-40/100 grippe patients--upon inadequate isolation techniques.[24]

Efforts to control hospital admissions of grippe patients were introduced early in the Fall of 1918, beginning with directives ordering hospitals to screen all influenza admissions. By October 14, demand for beds forced authorities to turn away all but cases with serious complications.[25] By October 22, Public Assistance was no longer accepting grippe patients;[26]

---

[21]Cruveilheir, 21.

[22]*Ibid.*

[23]*Ibid.*

[24]Lereboullet, 106, 111; cf. Fortineau, 80-81.

[25]Cruveilheir, 30.

[26]*Ibid.*

civilian authorities turned to the military who provided an additional 1,108 beds.[27]

On October 26, *Figaro* reported that Paris was suffering from a lack of medical personnel, due largely to the diversion of this resource to the military.[28] The situation was particularly acute in the 13th arrondisement, where only one physician served a largely indigent population.[29] Meanwhile, military physicians were encouraged to assist civilian physicians in the care of grippe patients.[30] Seeking further assistance, hospitals turned to the popular press to broadcast their need for volunteers on the grippe wards.[31] How many Parisiens responded to a crisis that would surely put them in jeopardy is unknown, but on November 7, 1918, the Director of Public Assistance issued a special thanks and praise for these brave volunteers.[32]

Until mid-November, Paris hospitals strained to accommodate grippe admissions. Then, just as hospitals could accept no more, grippe morbidity significantly dipped. "We cannot help but state with satisfaction," remarked a Paris physician, "that the grippe epidemic, which for the past months has been so deadly, is at this hour actually on decline."[33] This remarkable turn of events he credited to the cooperation between the civilian and military medical personnel.

While Paris daily life proceeded with but a slight nod to the grippe, the Paris medical community undertook a sustained response. The disease quickly became the subject of innumerable medical studies, publications, and academic presentations. In their reports in the popular press, the medical community supported the efficacy of prophylactic measures and initially

[27]*Ibid.*

[28]*Figaro*, Oct. 26, 1918; Cruveilheir, 30.

[29]*Ibid.*, 31.

[30]*Ibid.*, 30.

[31]*Figaro*, Oct. 23, 1918.

[32]Cruveilheir, 30.

[33]J. Castaigne, "Chronique," *Le Journal Médical Français*, 8 (1919): 51.

downplayed the severity of the epidemic.[34] As conveyed to the Paris public, the medical community appeared to exercise a measure of control and containment over this disease. Such an upbeat attitude could not be obtained from the medical literature, as will soon become apparent.

Although early in the epidemic grippe cases were not infrequently diagnosed as cholera and dysentery, physicians quickly concurred on the disease's clinical picture. The prodromal signs were general malaise, dizziness, lack of appetite, and chills. These were followed by fever, joint stiffness, syncope, headache, occipital and general myalgias; in addition, "the face was red, [and] a productive cough developed accompanied by a red pharynx and an characteristic porcelain glaze-like appearance of the tongue."[35] The grippe lasted from 2 to 3 days. The preponderance of patients were left with a lethargy and lingering cough; some developed depression. Twenty percent developed pulmonary complications. These cases were remarkable for the severity of symptoms and the rapidity with which certain forms progressed to death.

The French experience with the influenza epidemic of 1889-90 strongly influenced medical investigations into the grippe. French research on the late 19th century epidemic had used Koch's Postulates to implicate the causative role of the Pfeiffer bacillus. In 1918, many perceived the appearance of the grippe to be a variety of the 1889-90 epidemic; the Pfeiffer bacillus was once again implicated as the causative agent. Among the more frequently quoted advocates of this position, Dr. Arnold Netter had contributed to the isolation of the Pfeiffer bacillus during the 1889-90 epidemic. Reporting in November, 1918, Netter maintained that the grippe closely paralleled the earlier influenza epidemic in symptoms, contagious nature, and the role of the Pfeiffer bacillus.[36]

---

[34]Francis Heckel, "La Grippe, Son Traitement Préventif, Prophylaetique et Abortif," *L'Illustration* (Oct. 19, 1918), 373; Francis Heckel, "La Grippe Épidemique Actuelle," *L'Illustration* (Nov. 2, 1918), 425; *Figaro*, Oct. 11, 1918.

[35]Lereboullet, 33.

[36]Arnold Netter, "L'Épidemie d'Influenza de 1918," *Revue d'Hygiène et de Police Sanitaire*, 40 (1918): 543-553.

His confident position was corroborated by the results of research conducted in France, England, and Germany, but encountered challenges from reports that pure samples of the Pfeiffer bacillus were impossible to obtain. To these findings, Netter argued that, while "the pneumococci, streptococci, etc., are not specific agents of the influenza, they play an important role in its complications."[37] Their irritating action provides the appropriate, if not necessary substratum for the Pfeiffer bacillus. In further support of his position, Netter argued that failure to culture the Pfeiffer bacillus in grippe patients did not refute his findings; rather, it indicated faulty sampling techniques and repeated samples would eliminate these negative findings.[38]

Despite the arguments of Netter and other supporters of the 1889-90 parallel, bacterial origins of grippe remained unestablished,[39] although medical consensus agreed on the bacterial causes of the dreaded pulmonary complications. In England, a vaccine against these agents was in use by early fall, 1918.[40] French efforts resulted in vaccine preparation by late fall, 1918.[41]

Less agreement was reached on the role of the so-called filterable viruses. In 1899, French researchers had described a "microbe of peripneumonia" which could not be seen microscopically and was remarkable for its ability to pass through a porcelain filter.[42] Suspicion of the role of these filterable viruses in the grippe emerged early in the epidemic and generated studies using human and animal subjects. The work of Charles

---

[37]*Ibid.*, 547.

[38]*Ibid.*, 548.

[39]Lereboullet, 22; Castaigne, 14; Louis Renon, "La Thérapeutique Moderne de la Grippe," *Le Journal Médical Français*, 8 (1919): 32.

[40]Renon, 33.

[41]Lereboullet, 109.

[42]D. Roussy, "Nature et Modes d'Action de l'Agent Pathogène Infectieux de la Grippe ou Influenza," *Revue d'Hygiène et de Police Sanitaire*, 41 (1919): 114.

Nicolle and Charles LeBailly, French physicians, was the most frequently cited of these efforts.

Speaking to the Academy of Science on October 14, 1918, Nicolle and LeBailly described the methods by which they isolated the virus and reproduced the grippe in monkeys that had been injected with the viral serum.[43] Describing the specific steps taken to obtain the viral serum, Nicolle and LeBailly then explained that they deposited the viral filtrant onto the monkeys' conjunctiva and nasal mucosa; flu-like symptoms subsequently developed. The viral serum was also used to induce grippe experimentally in human subjects. In this case, the filtrant injected under the skin purportedly gave rise to flu-like symptoms while that injected into the veins had no results.

Dujarric de la Rivière, who also inoculated human subjects subcutaneously with viral substrate, offered contemporary corroboration of Nicolle and LeBailly's investigations.[44] He reportedly produced flu-like symptoms with this method. Tantalizing observations that grippe resembled certain flu-like diseases in swine were presented at this time,[45] but speculation on a possible connection between influenza in man and animals, however, centered on the horse.[46]

Critics of Nicolle and LeBailly's conclusions argued that the experiments failed to control for opportunistic infections with grippe. Monkeys, they further argued, were highly susceptible to a wide spectrum of upper respiratory illnesses, and thus, undesirable subjects. Despite these objections, the attempts to ascertain a viral cause of grippe proceeded in

---

[43]Charles Nicolle and Charles LeBailly, "Recherches Experimentales sur la Grippe," *Annales de l'Institut Pasteur*, 33 (1919): 395-402; cf. Report of findings in *Figaro*, Oct. 15, 1918.

[44]Dujarric de la Rivière, "La Grippe Est-Elle un Maladie à Virus Filtrant?" *C.R. Académie des Sciences*, 167 (1918): 606.

[45]Lereboullet, 96.

[46]*Ibid.*, 96-97; Francis Heckel, "Aurons-Nous la Grippe? et Pourquoi Nous l'Avons Eue," *L'Illustration*, (Nov. 22, 1919): 154; A. Orticone et L. Barbie, "La Pandemie Grippale de 1918. Relations de la Grippe Humaine avec certaines Epizooties Animales," *Revue d'Hygiène et de Police Sanitaire*, 41 (1919): 386-428; Beveridge, 56-57.

France and on an international scale. These investigations developed more rigorous controls of experimental subjects and increased the sampling sizes, another attempt to counter the virus critics. The final breakthrough came in 1928, too late to assist with the grippe although clearly informed by investigations this epidemic and encouraged.[47]

Prophylactic measures advanced for grippe were based upon the realization that it was a highly contagious airborne disease. On October 8, 1918, the Under Secretary of State to the Minister of War approached the Academy of Medicine for urgent assistance in halting the spread of the grippe.[48] Meanwhile, the views of the French physician Trillat, who maintained that air supported and nourished grippe germs, intensified concerns over the disease's contagious nature.[49] Physicians urged the avoidance of crowds and other places where contact with grippe victims was probable. They advised masks for persons working with grippe patients and suggested droplets placed inside the nose as another means of avoiding the infection.[50] Arsenic was touted as a preventative measure.[51] *L'Illustration* told its readers that persons treated with arsenic and regularly exposed to the grippe suffered no infection.[52]

Uncertain about the actual cause, physicians treated the disease symptomatically. Treatment preferences varied among physicians and even, within a given practice, among patients, but generally included one or more of the medications summarized by Louis Renon, Professor, Faculty of Paris, and physician, Necker Hospital. Renon stated that seven treatment

---

[47]cf. *Ibid.*, 2-4.

[48]Report of the Academy of Medicine Oct. 8, 1918, *La Presse Médicale*, 26 (1918): 532.

[49]Heckel, "Aurons-Nous la Grippe?," 426.

[50]Heckel,"La Grippe. Son Traitement. . .," 373.

[51]Renon, 37.

[52]Heckel, "La Grippe. Son Traitement. . .," 373. Robert Koch's study of the restraining influence of arsenic solution on the growth of anthrax bacilli demonstrated the antiseptic properties of arsenic. See C. Binz, *Lecture on Pharmacology for Practitioners and Students*, trans. by P.W. Latham, Vol. 11 (London, 1897): 91.

modalities had become standard in treating the grippe. They included antipyretics, metallic solutions, stimulants, antiseptics, biological medicine (vaccines), and revulsions. Renon maintained that this diversity of treatment represented therapeutic uncertainty. The simple grippe "has a natural tendency to cure itself," he noted, while the severe cases often resist attempts at any and all therapeutic intervention.[53]

Among the antipyretics, quinine salts and powder, the latter mixed with coffee, were popularly used. Renon could not account for the "vogue of quinine medication," as he found it of no benefit for his patients.[54] Aspirin also exhibited counter-indications, including profuse sweating and weakness. On the antipyretics as a whole, Renon cautioned that their effect was ephemeral. "The often give the illusion of of resolution. . . the colloidal medications merit greater attention."[55]

The treatment value of the colloids was inconclusive, Renon acknowledged, yet he noted that they were widely applied to combat the grippe. Colloids of gold, silver, tin, rhodium, and other metallics were injected intravenously or intramuscularly. Renon cautioned that intravenous injections were "a little brutal;"[56] he preferred rhodium injected intramuscularly. Later accounts underlined the harsh nature of these treatments and questioned their efficacy.[57]

Stimulants commonly used included acetate of ammonia, caffeine, and alcohol, administered orally, and camphor, strychnine, and arsenic, administered intravenously. Without explaining their efficacy, Renon maintained that these treatments "are necessary in the grippe."[58]

---

[53]Renon, 35.

[54]*Ibid.*

[55]*Ibid.*

[56]*Ibid.*, 34.

[57]Lereboullet, 120.

[58]Renon, 36.

Antiseptics were also accepted treatments. Renon cited compounds that provided either weak bacterio-static action, as in the case of methalyine blue, or, as tropines, promoted weak bronchial relaxation and inhibited secretions. He also suggested the antiseptic treatment of choice for pneumonia in horses, although he noted that some regarded it with great scepticism.

Renon advised regular administration of adrenaline compound as adjuncts to the stimulants. Low blood pressure (specific indications not offered) was indication for their use. He classified this treatment as "*mèdication opothérapique*," referring to a therapy that many believed assisted the organs of defense, assumed to be the thyroid and the adrenals.[59]

While Renon largely avoided treatment rationales, the stimulants that he described shared an underlying therapeutic imperative to arouse the patient's defenses. Stimulants, irritants, "*opothérapie*" were believed to be "powerful aides that nobly augmented the organism's means of defense."[60] The rationale for these remedies rested largely upon the prevailing commitment to heroic medicine; this worked on the assumption that the stronger the intervention, the more the body's defenses will be stimulated to react. Agents that stimulated the sympathetic nervous system, and specifically the adrenals, were treatments of choice. Explaining this approach, Dr. Heckel informed readers of *L'Illustration* that success in treating grippe was achieved much like success on the battlefield: it required measures that seized the initiative from the enemy.[61]

When other stimulants failed, heroic medicine resorted to the ancient revulsive treatments of bleeding and scarification.[62] Indeed, Renon held that bleeding was essential in the treatment of all grippe cases. Others advised its use primarily in cases of pulmonary edema secondary to grippe. Most

---

59*cf.* Heckel, "La Grippe. Son Traitement. . .," 373.

60H. Paillard, "Remarques Cliniques et Methodes Thérapeutiques dans la Grippe," *Le Journal Médical Français*, 8 (1919): 44.

61Heckel, "Nouvelles Observations. . .," 449.

62The third pillar of ancient treatments--purging--was not advised. See Lereboullet, 119.

believed it was counterindicated in cases of extreme malaise, which further depletion of resources would aggravate. In these latter instances, scarification was an adequate substitute.

This took two forms: Renon described the application of a large amount of cupping--6 to 10 applications--daily. The other, more intense procedure was called the "fixed abscess." It was indicated in cases with grim prognosis, particularly septicemias and bronchial pneumonias. In his article, "The Technique of the Fixed Abscess in Grippe," the physician Paillard shared his personal experience with this therapy. He acknowledged that some disputed its efficacy,[63] but he found it "to obtain remarkable and even unhoped for results"[64] in treating grippe.

Injecting turpentine subcutaneously into the thigh provoked the abscess. Follow-up treatment involved maintaining asepsis by lancing and taking repeated cultures to maintain asepsis. When the abscess became purulent, the patient should become afebrile. Paillard noted that the abscess, when used in conjunction with surgical interventions in septicemias, aided in a favorable outcome.

Renon did not give the "biological medicines," or vaccines, his unqualified support. "Their curative action is difficult to judge, [he explained] because of the natural tendency of uncomplicated cases to resolve spontaneously and the possibility that even the most grave will improve, regardless of what treatments are employed."[65] He noted, however, that vaccines produce few untoward complications and that, in fact, they have been used in grave cases and have had favorable outcomes. Relative to antipneumonic serum, which had recently been developed, they were decidedly inferior.

Of the available vaccines, Renon discussed the vaccine developed in England which protected against the Pfeiffer bacillus, pneumococcus and

---

[63]cf. *Ibid.*, 127.

[64]H. Paillard, "Technique de l'Abcès de Fixation dans la Grippe," *Le Journal Médical Français*, 8 (1919): 47.

[65]Renon, 37.

streptococcus, and the vaccine developed by M. Depede, which was composed of pneumococcus, enterococcus, and streptococcus. Writing on the grippe in 1926, Dr. Pierre Lereboullet noted that the polyvalent vaccines were directed against the most dangerous aspect of the grippe--the secondary complications--and produced disappointing therapeutic results.[66]

Seriotherapy, of which Renon was strong advocate, included the antipneumococcus serum developed at the Pasteur Institute. Renon claimed to have used it in cases where pneumococcus were present and reported favorable resolution of symptoms in each case.[67]

The efficacy of serum developed from the blood of former grippe patients was announced early in October, 1918,[68] and was widely recognized as beneficial. Similarly positive results had been obtained from serums developed from convalescing measles and scarlet fever patients. Renon maintained that the serum, when administered early in the disease, was nearly uniformly efficacious; administered after the fifth day of infection, it was ineffective.[69] The inability to provide large enough quantities and safe storage methods to meet the demand for this effective therapy prevented its wide-spread use.

France was divided into sanitary districts headed by sanitary commissions that consulted with local medical and public health professionals for policy development. Within the municipalities, elected officials, usually the mayor, initiated public health measures or enacted those advised by his sanitary region. The mayor's action proceeded with the approval of his departmental assemblies and the cooperation of the prefect of police, who enforced public health edicts. The Minister of the Interior oversaw this loose organization. The fall appearance of the grippe elicited a formal declaration from this high office. Issued on September 18, 1918, the

---

[66]Lereboullet, 115.

[67]Renon, 38.

[68]H. Violle, "Pandémie de la Grippe," *La Presse Médicale*, 26 (1918): 527.

[69]*cf.* Lereboullet, 121.

declaration warned that the disease was dangerous and offered measures to contain it.

Localities were advised to take appropriate steps to assure accurate epidemiological records. They were urged to cooperate with regional sanitary personnel in implementing prophylactic measures, the most important of these being disinfection. Isolation of grippe patients was another measure considered; hospitalization was advised, although the burden to hospitals presented by persons dislocated by the war was recognized. The circular also addressed the shortage of civilian physicians; as a temporary solution, prefects were to request relief physicians from their regional sanitary director. The Minister's office was to be notified if these efforts failed. Finally, restraints on public gatherings were presented but only as a possibility, should the epidemic worsen. No restraints could be implemented without the prior approval of appropriate officials within the Minister of Interior's Office.[70]

Timely in its warning, the circular advanced standard measures against infectious disease, namely isolation and disinfection. It also addressed significant shortcomings in health care delivery and recognized the war's drain upon medical resources as the more drastic of these. In addition, it hinted at an endemic weakness in the French public health system: physicians' resistance to government interference. Physician opposition to the *declaration obligatoire*, that legally required them to report infectious disease, severely hampered public health efforts to establish morbidity counts and epidemiological patterns during epidemics. This imposed information gap also stymied efforts to stem spread of contagion through disinfection of private homes.[71]

Physicians insisted that the *declaration obligatoire* interfered with the doctor-patient relationship and forced them to violate patient confidence.

---

[70]France, "Circulaire du Ministre de l'Intérieur."

[71]For a discussion of French physician resistance to reporting contagious disease, see Ann-Louise Shapiro, "Private Rights, Public Interest, and Professional Jurisdiction: The French Public Health Law of 1902," *Bulletin of the History of Medicine*, 54 (1980): 4-22; *cf.* Daniel M. Fox. "Social Policy and City Politics: Tuberculosis Reporting in New York, 1889-1900," *Bulletin of the History of Medicine*, 49 (1975): 169-195.

Such betrayal, physicians further argued, also had untoward consequences for the patient and his family: jobs were lost, credit vanished, and social standing was severely threatened. The reporting physician faced similar consequences: his practice suffered from word of mouth warning.

In Paris, resistance to the *declaration obligatoire* exacerbated a town-gown controversy. Reacting to opposition within the private practice sphere, the Academy of Medicine in July, 1913, voted 51 to 34 in favor of the *declaration obligatoire*.[72] In October, 1918, as the influenza pandemic gathered speed, an organization of Paris physicians soundly rejected the *declaration obligatoire* and refused to recognize its legal status.[73] Tempers flared in the Spring of 1919, in the waning days of the grippe, as the Academy of Medicine mounted a campaign to include tuberculosis within the *declaration obligatoire*. In 1902, this disease had been removed from the list of reportable diseases because of strong physician opposition.[74] The spokesman for the opposition in 1919 likened reporting a patient's tuberculosis to the treason of Judas.[75]

The persistence of a general resistance to the *declaration obligatoire* distorted the official public health view of grippe morbidity and mortality in Paris. Undoubtedly it also reduced incidence of disinfection. While a standard preventive measure, disinfection was not regarded as effective by all sectors of the medical community.[76] Ideally, disinfection of private homes involved the entire house and all household goods. Practically, it was often incomplete and without necessary follow-up. Actually, the process was intrusive, disruptive, and humiliating. Physicians rationalized that ignoring the *declaration obligatoire* was in their patients' best interest. Further supporting this argument, they contended that their actions did not unduly

---

[72] *Figaro*, April 2, 1919.

[73] *Ibid.*

[74] Shapiro, 18.

[75] *Figaro*, April 2, 1919.

[76] Lereboullet, 104.

harm society, as the public health merits of disinfection procedures were dubious.[77]

In Paris, the splintering of governmental powers further hampered public health efforts. Paris had two separate prefects enforcing public health measures, the Prefect of Police and the Prefect of the Seine. Effective implementation of measures against the grippe depended upon the coordination and cooperation of these two offices,[78] yet, neither had the power to impose procedures.[79]

In early October, 1918, the 16th Commission of Municipal Councils visited Paris to examine the state of sanitation of the city and suburbs in the wake of the ongoing epidemic of dysentery.[80] At this time, the council observed that the grippe was far less lethal than the grippe of 1889-90; they advised, however, that measures against it should be taken.[81] The disinfection procedures advised by the Commission and the Declaration of September 18, 1918, were more successfully implemented in the larger cities like Paris that had the advantage of trained personnel and appropriate equipment. On October 9, 1918, the Commission's advice was implemented and Paris officials expressed confidence that all measures of precaution against the grippe had been taken.[82] The epidemic, however, was still in its early phase.

On October 13, 1918, announcement of further measures to disinfect public places in Paris was reported in *Figaro*. A report of October 17

---

[77]For a discussion of physician opposition to disinfection, see Dr. Guy-Laroche and M. Lauby, "Étude sur le Reorganisation des Services d'Hygiène en France," *Revue d'Hygiène et de Police Sanitaire*, 41 (1919): 1003-1209 and Leon Bernard, "Sur le Projet de Revision de la Loi du 15 Fevrier 1902 sur la Protection de la Santé Publique," *Annales d'Hygiène Publique et de Médecine Legale*, 35 (1921): 65-160.

[78]Bernard, 80-81.

[79]Shapiro, 23.

[80]*Figaro*, Oct. 9, 1918.

[81]*Ibid.*

[82]*Ibid.*

declared that the Paris schools were disinfected.[83] *L'Illustration* reported that the government was requiring disinfection of private homes of persons with the grippe and was preparing to disinfect trains; measures to separate civilian travelers from military travelers were also reported.[84] This last measure recognized the role of the returning soldier in communicating the grippe to French civilians.

On Thursday, October 17, 1918, *Figaro* carried the report of the Academy of Medicine meeting of the previous Monday. Alarm over the rapidly increasing number of grippe cases was apparent. The easy transmissibility of the disease was iterated and the necessity of isolation, disinfection, and avoidance of public places emphasized. The *Municipal Bulletin* was quoted as reporting 1,445 deaths for the week, against 989 the week before and an average of 721 for the season.[85] On October 26, as the number of grippe cases soared, *Figaro* carried the medical community's dissatisfaction with the government's laissez-faire policy. Doctors complained about the diversion of medical resources to the military and the scarcity of disinfectants and medicines. And, they reproached the government for failing to restrict public gatherings.[86] Lyon had implemented such a restriction, they noted, but Paris officials had rejected it early in the epidemic.[87]

Calls for a reorganization of the national public hygiene administration followed in the wake of the grippe epidemic and underscored the shortcomings of a system that had been constructed out of patchwork legislation since the emergence of the Paris Health Council in 1802.[88]

[83]*Ibid.*, Oct. 17, 1918.

[84]Heckel, "La Grippe. Son Traitement. . .," 373.

[85]*Figaro*, Oct. 17, 1918.

[86]*Ibid.*, Oct. 26, 1918.

[87]*Ibid.*

[88]For a discussion of this Council and its importance to the development of public health in France, see Ann Fowler LeBerge, "The Paris Health Council, 1802-1848," *Bulletin of the History of Medicine*, 49 (1975): 339-52.

Directives for change, however, came not from experience with the grippe, but from lessons learned from the Rockefeller Commission's recent success in establishing effective public health measures against tuberculosis in France. The impetus was provided by the devastation and dislocation of the war; the immediate health needs of so many in such critical times compelled an efficient, effective public health organization. In 1919, pronouncements of the new public health organization omitted the grippe from the list of diseases cited as major public health concerns.[89] One year after the disease had claimed so many victims, it was no longer a pressing memory.

In Paris, indications of major concern about the grippe emerged largely from the medical community. In this arena, the disease had the salutary effect of encouraging research into filterable viruses, recently discovered and implicated in influenza, while broadening medicine's understanding of the action of bacteria in secondary infection. Actively involved in discovering the grippe's cause and directing treatments for its cure, the medical community provided the substantive response to this disease.

Responses from other sectors of the Paris community were diluted by the overriding war effort and diverted by the city's policy of not alarming the public with intrusive public health measures. Little of Paris' daily life or night time entertainments was curtailed by the disease. Whatever public alarm may have been developing in October, as grippe mortality climbed, was relieved by the fortunately brief duration of this acute phase. Fragmented public health measures largely escaped public opprobrium, as the depleting war effort received the blame for the grippe's ravages. Buoyed by the promise of Versailles and weary of mortality statistics, Paris quietly endured the brief battle with the grippe and consigned its memory to the families of its unfortunate victims and to medicine.

---

[89]Guy-Laroche et M. Lauby, 1003; *Figaro*, April 27, 1919; George Vitoux, "Congrès Interallié d'Hygiène Sociale Pour la Reconstruction des Régions Dévastées par la Guerre," *Revue d'Hygiène et Police Sanitaire*, 41 (1919): 573.

Chapter 5: Manchester

Fred R. van Hartesveldt

To Englishmen inured by three and a half years of butcher's bills from the Western Front, reports in the spring of 1918 of an influenza pandemic were hardly bone chilling. As the ailment touched Africa, the United States, and the Continent, where it unfairly became known as "Spanish Flu," the English paid little attention, and since the early version was comparatively mild, this was hardly unreasonable. The malady was not in its usual form, however, for by mid-1919 it would take more than 200,000 lives in the British Isles.

Arriving in late June, the pandemic swept over Britain in three waves. The first in the summer of 1918 was the most infectious and the least deadly, killing, by official count, only 17,500. The second came in the winter of 1918 leaving 115,000 dead, and the third arrived early in 1919 to kill another 51,000. Even the Ministry of Health, which collected these figures after the fact, conceded that they are estimates. Due to confused diagnoses, inadequate record keeping, and failure to make influenza reportable until well into the third wave, they are certainly low estimates. More important for a disease with relative low mortality is the case-rate figure. Unfortunately cases were not counted systematically. Estimates made from surveys taken after the final wave was gone vary from about 5% to something over 20% of the population being ill. Even if the lower figure is accepted, there were more than three and one-half million cases in England and Wales in forty-six weeks.[1] The weakness of such estimates is made clear by the report of a London Medical Officer of Health, who was one of very few to follow up on fatalities. He found that of 208 fatal cases, 131 or 62.98% had no contact with a health care professional while ill.[2] Fatalities, although certainly misdiagnosed at times, were reported, but if significantly more than half of those cases serious enough to cause death went unattended other than by friends and relatives, one must wonder how many less serious cases were not reported in any way. Block surveys that were done do not seem to have been either systematic or random samples, hence the author's opinion that official estimates are substantially low.

Manchester and neighboring Salford--the two, divided by the river Irwell, were connected by a dozen bridges at the time of the pandemic--are part of the industrial region of southeastern Lancashire. Cotton, cloth and coal were particularly important among the products of the region, and thanks to their river and canal connections, Manchester and Salford offered port services to the whole area. The initial years of the 20th century were a time of rapid human and physical growth in these cities, but by the time of the war they had stabilized. The estimated populations of the two in 1918 were Manchester 770,248 and Salford 209,274. About ten years after the war, the population of the two cities comprised one fortieth of the total population of Great Britain.[3] The concentration of economic development and population and unified health administration (unlike London) make

---

[1]Ministry of Health, *Reports on Public Health and Medical Subjects*. No. 4: *Report on the Pandemic of Influenza, 1918-19* (London, 1920), 548, 557. Hereafter Ministry of Health, *Report on the Pandemic.*

[2]Metropolitan Borough of St. Pancras, *Annual Report of Medical Officer of Health for 1918* (London, 1919), 42.

[3]E.M. Brockbank (ed.), *The Book of Manchester and Salford* (Manchester, n.d.), 1, 199, 207; Manchester, *Annual Report of Medical Officer of Health for 1918* (Manchester, 1919), 1 (Hereafter Manchester, *1918 Report*); Salford, *Annual Report of Medical Officer of Health of 1918* (Salford, 1918), 11. (Hereafter Salford, *1918 Report.*) These reports were seen in the Local Collection of the Manchester Central Library. (Hereafter Central Lib.) The Manchester population estimate is significantly higher than that made by the Registrar General. See *Annual Report of the Registrar General of Births Deaths and Marriages in England and Wales for 1917-18*, (London, 1919), 20.

Manchester--with some Salford data included--an excellent focus for a case study of the pandemic's impact in Britain.

In 1918 the influenza mortality rate for the country was 3.13 and for Manchester 2.71 per 1000 population. In 1919 the Manchester rate fell to 2.0. Manchester was, then, somewhat less severely hit than the country as a whole (Overall it ranked 26th among country boroughs and Salford 29th), however, its rates in 1891 and 1892, the peak of the preceding pandemic, were .76 and .32 respectively. No recorded mortality rate between 1913 and 1919 was higher than the 1918 influenza figure, and in 1918 for the first time since records had been kept, the Manchester death-rate approached the birth-rate.[4] The impact of the pandemic compared to other common causes of death can be seen in Table 5.1. Influenza deaths comprised 15.04% of deaths in Salford in 1918 and 12.6% in 1919. The corresponding figures for Manchester are 17.2% and 10.38% for 1918-19 and 3.6% and 1.2% in 1891 and 1892.[5]

Tables 5.2 and 5.3 illustrate, for the country and Manchester, one of the highly unusual aspects of the 1918-19 pandemic. It struck most severely at people in their mid-twenties to mid-fifties--middle-aged by the standards of the day. In Salford, for instance, 61.87% of the deaths during the first wave were of people 25 to 55 years of age.[6] Normally the very young and very old, particularly the latter, are the the most badly affected by influenza.

---

[4]Registrar General, *Supplement to the Eighty-First Annual Report of Births, Deaths, and Marriages in England and Wales. Report on the Mortality from Influenza in England and Wales During the Epidemic of 1918-19* (London, 1920), 3, 7; Manchester, *1918 Report*, 2, 25; Salford, *1918 Report*, 16-17; John Tatham, Medical Officer of Health, *Report on the Health of Greater Manchester 1891-93* (Manchester, 1894), 65--Table 12.

[5]Manchester, *1918 Report*, 160--Table A; *Ibid.* for 1919, 262-Table A; Salford, *1918 Report*, 14--Table M4; *Ibid.* for 1919, 16-Table M4; Tatham, 83-94.

[6]Salford, *1918 Report*, 24.

Table 5.1

Chief Causes of Death in Manchester

	1915	*1916*	*1917*	*1918*	*1919*	*1920*
Tuberculosis of the Lungs	1315	1238	1196	1103	951	868
Tuberculosis not of the Lungs	313	348	359	287	237	220
Heart Disease	1163	1025	947	920	1050	1076
Cerebral Hemor-rhage, Apoplexy, Hemiplegia	543	553	604	503	483	462
Pneumonia	1089	944	929	1421	977	919
Bronchitis	1278	1207	1097	1053	1277	1193
Digestive Organs	517	454	396	360	397	373
Atrophy, Debility	277	164	155	153	144	245
Old Age	520	429	439	413	464	408
Premature Birth	350	317	262	280	324	378
Nephritis and Bright's Disease	369	335	307	275	275	283
Brain Inflamation	98	74	76	77	65	65
Diarrhea and Dysentery	488	313	279	147	172	250
Measles, Scarlet Fever, Whopping Cough, Diptheria	705	581	404	575	211	407
Influenza	136	133	98	2096	1127	229
Malignant Disease	775	794	770	806	875	836

Source: Annual Reports of Manchester Medical Officer of Health, 1919, 2--Table 1 and 1920, 16--Table 5.

The impact of the disease in this case was thus worsened by the loss of disproportionate numbers at the most productive ages. The odd pattern of mortality distribution by age is typical of the world's experience in 1918-19. Table 5.3 provides a comparison with the most recent prior pandemic and to 1920, the year following the pandemic. The odd pattern existed for males as well as females, eliminating the possibility that it was produced by the population displacement due to men being away in service. It seems largely confined to the 1918-1919 outbreak (though there was some hint of it in the early 1890s), but no explanation has been found. Despite many efforts to find other patterns--occupation, wealth, living conditions--no clear ones have emerged.[7]

Table 5.2

Deaths By Age
Epidemic of 1918-19 Compared to that of 1890-91

	Age Groups					
	0-9	*10-19*	*20-34*	*35-54*	*55-74*	*75-*
1890	885	237	621	1,175	1,330	516
1891	2,733	658	1,759	4,065	6,091	2,171
Total 1890-91	3,618	895	2,398	5,230	7,421	2,687
Total 1918-19	26,667	16,197	52,491	34,645	20,228	4,209

Source: Registrar General, *Report on the mortality from Influenza in England and Wales During the Epidemic of 1918-19*, Supplement to the Eighty-first Report, CMD 700 (London, 1920), 32--Table XV; Local Government Board, *Further Report and Report and Papers on Epidemic Influenza, 1889-92*, CMD 7051 (London, 1893), 1-2, 25.

---

[7]Ministry of Health, *Report on the Pandemic*, 533, 556.

The Medical Officer of Health (MOH) in Manchester in 1918 was James Niven, who had held the office since 1894. A Scotsman who had studied at St. Thomas's Hospital, Niven had a solid reputation for work concerning infectious diseases and sanitation before coming to Manchester. During his 28 year tenure the Manchester death-rate--which in 1898 at 24.80 was third highest for the thirty-three great towns--was halved, the city got its first isolation hospital (Monsall), and sanitation and pollution problems were generally ameliorated, although in 1915 nearly half of the households still lacked flush toilets.[8] Mancunians were in much better hands as far as getting a productive response to the pandemic than most of the nation.

Table 5.3

Manchester Influenza Mortality by Age
(per 1000 Population)

	All	0-1	1-4	5-14	15-24	25-44	45-64	65-
1891	.69	.03	.03	.01	.04	.18	.24	.16
1892	.28	.02	.02	.02	.02	.07	.09	.05
1917	.15	.01	.01	.01	.00	.02	.06	.05
1918	3.15	.09	.37	.33	.42	1.39	.65	.23
1919	1.69	.06	.14	.09	.18	.56	.42	.25
1920	.34	.02	.01	.01	.04	.09	.11	.06

Source: John Tatham, *Report on the Health of Greater Manchester, 1891-93* (Manchester, 1894), 83-84--Table B; *Annual Report of Medical Officer of Health for Manchester, 1917* (Manchester, 1918), 135--Table A; *Ibid.* for 1918, 164-65--Tables B & C.

[8]Willis J. Elwood and A. Felicite Tuxford (eds.), *Some Manchester Doctors* (Manchester, 1984), 98-100; Shena D. Simon, *A Century of City Government: Manchester 1838-1938* (London, 1938), 167; Arthur Redford with Ina Stafford Russell, *The History of Local Government in Manchester* Vol. 3: *The Last Half Century* (London, 1940), 315.

Before 1914, Victorian individualism and hostility to collective action had not yet succumbed to "war socialism." The power of local authorities to require use of such things as ambulance and disinfection services, which the Public Health Act of 1875 allowed them to provide, was restricted to notifiable diseases i.e. those that had to be reported to the government. The MOH was originally mostly a public health administrative officer, but in ts

Manchester, Niven had, by 1918, begun a voluntary notification of tuberculosis (1899), started a Midwives Supervising Committee (1904), created a staff of health visitors based on the Ladies' Public Health Society (1908), established municipal control of six welfare centers of the School for Mothers (1915), started a scheme for treating venereal disease (1917), and made other reforms. In addition to the various sanitary improvements, public education in connection with public health was widespread thanks to the Manchester and Salford Sanitary Association, with key leadership from Arthur Ransome.[9] War made health harder to maintain, and 1918 saw the introduction of food rationing, rapidly rising fuel prices, and an unusually cold winter.[10] Although the influenza was no respecter of reforms, the experience of both officials and citizenry with an active public health program made efforts to deal with the pandemic much easier to establish.

The first wave of flu, late June to early August, was mostly an annoyance with a variety of services disrupted by workers absent due to illness. June 28, the tramways reported 250 absentees, more than three times the normal rate; the number rose to 760 ten days later. Service was much reduced. By mid-July, 39,255 school children had been reported ill, and a number of elementary schools were closed. Although the death-rate remained relatively low, the press reported that grave diggers were hard pressed. Niven met the arrival of the disease with a leaflet of advice including bed rest, wearing muslin masks, and the use of a vaccine upon the

---

[9]James Niven, *Observations on the History of Public Health Effort in Manchester* (Manchester and London, 1923), 14, 202; Jeanne L. Brand, *Doctors and the State: The Medical Profession and Government Action in Public Health, 1870-1912* (Baltimore, 1965), 152; Anthony S. Wohl, *Endangered Lives: Public Health in Victorian England* (Cambridge, MA, 1983), 68-70, 97-98.

[10](Manchester) *Evening Chronicle*, January 28, 1919; (Salford) *Reporter*, June 28, Sept. 7, 1918, Jan. 4, 1919.

recommendation of a physician. Posters with the same advice were placed around town, and the newspapers gave it prominence as well. Although many requests for disinfection of buildings were made to the authorities, only rarely were municipal resources provided, but advice about disinfectants was freely given. Dr. Niven recommended that even in mild cases the victim should stay away from groups for ten days and in severe cases he should stay home for three weeks.[11] Had the experience of wave one been the pattern for the entire outbreak, the 1918-19 pandemic would have been remembered as just an unusually harsh example of the recurring cycle of influenza. The arrival of the second wave soon changed the attitude to one of real concern.

The next outbreak began, according to Niven, on October 19, and although it proved somewhat less widespread than the first, it was much more deadly. In the week ending November 30, there were 383 deaths. Burial took a fortnight, if a coffin could be found.[12] Niven remarked that it was "imperative that the War Office. . . send skilled coffin-makers back to the workshop without delay."[13] Niven also urged that people forego elaborate funerals and recommended cremation. With the help of a detachment of the Labor Corps of the Western Command of the Royal Army to dig graves, the worst of the second wave was handled. The third wave, early in 1919, was worse in Manchester than in most of the rest of the country and also required outside laborers as grave diggers. Fortunately, the peak of 122 deaths in the week ending March 8, 1919, was much lower than that of the fall.[14]

During the second and third waves advice continued to pour out to the populace, but direct action to prevent infection was also taken. The schools were closed in each wave in hopes of limiting exposure, with the children being out from November 29 to January 6.[15] There were concerns

[11]Ministry of Health, *Report on the Pandemic*, 472-474. See also Manchester, *1918 Report*, 34; *Manchester Guardian*, June 28, 1918; (Manchester) *Evening Chronicle*, July 2, July 8, 1918.

[12]Ministry of Health, *Report on the Pandemic*, 474-77.

[13]*Manchester Guardian*, Nov. 30, 1918.

[14](Salford) *Reporter*, March 22, 1919.

[15]*Manchester Guardian*, Nov. 29, 1918; (Salford) *Reporter*, Nov. 30, 1918.

that the children would simply gather together in cinemas and other places of entertainment if not in school. Some people urged that schools be kept open unless there were simply no teachers well enough to maintain them to keep children off the streets while parents worked or were ill. The Local Government Board in London issued regulations limiting theaters to no more than three hours continuous entertainment followed by thirty minute intermissions during which the building was to be thoroughly ventilated. These regulations were strictly enforced in Manchester.[16] Although not national policy, in Manchester those under fourteen were not admitted at all. In response to urging that such establishments be closed, the mayor of Salford remarked that they would be if he had the power to do so. Although in some places such restrictions were resisted by owners, no such problems were reported in Manchester, except for some Sunday Schools which persisted in meeting as usual. Warnings seem to have little effect, however, for attendance at moving pictures did not decline during the pandemic.[17]

While resting if ill and avoiding crowds were useful ideas, other recommendations for dealing with the "Spanish Flu" were largely worthless. The wearing of muslin or gauze masks over the nose and mouth was common in the United States, but Niven was unusual in urging it in England. People might be willing to go to bed, disinfect homes and businesses, gargle with approved disinfectants, even use the suggested vaccine, but "women," remarked the *Evening Chronicle*, "are not going to wear ugly masks."[18] In fact few Mancunians, male or female, bothered, and as is now known, the virus is too small to be stopped by any cloth. The vaccine was of no more use than the masks. Although the exact formula varied from version to version, Niven, like others, advocated a composition of Pfeiffer's bacillus (regarded since the 1890s as the causal agent of influenza), pneumonococci, and

---

[16] *Ibid.*, Nov. 9, 1918; *Manchester Guardian*, Nov. 21, 1918; (Manchester) *Evening Chronicle*, Feb. 14, Feb. 27, 1919.

[17] (Salford) *Reporter*, Nov. 2, 1918; Manchester, *1918 Report*, 34; *Manchester Guardian*, Nov. 26, 1918; (Manchester) *Evening Chronicle*, March 1, 1919.

[18] *Ibid.*, Feb. 18, 1919. See also (Salford) *Reporter*, Dec. 11, 1918; *Manchester Guardian*, Feb. 14, 1919.

streptococci. The latter were added since Pfeiffer's bacillus was not always found in cases of influenza and they often were.[19]

Unlike many of his colleagues, James Niven not only recognized the medical danger but also acted to help individuals in need of non-medical support. Efforts were undertaken through the city Public Health Committee to provide domestic help where needed, especially when neighbors and relatives were too ill or frightened to enter the houses of the sick. Unfortunately, such help, especially qualified nurses, was at a premium. Despite much good will the Manchester and Salford District Nursing Association reported that due to much illness in the ranks of its members only a few were available; those who could, however, often gave generously of time day and night.[20] On December 4, all of the health visitors were shifted to visiting and caring for those suffering from influenza. The number of special investigations had been zero in 1916 and 149 in 1917, but it rose to 2,252 in 1918 and 5,636 in 1919.[21] Care was taken to ensure that every house where there was a fatality was visited and as many others as possible. Part of a donation of coal from December, 1916, remained and was used to help ease suffering. Of 970 requests for coal sanctioned--a means test was required--in 1918, 143 were specifically in response to the pandemic. In 1919, 290 applications were sanctioned with 110 arising from influenza.[22] Additional help in the form of milk, nursing, and whiskey--the most frequently prescribed medication for influenza in England--was given in

---

[19]For the formula adopted by the Ministry of Health see Ministry of Health, *Report on the Pandemic*, XX. This is typical although ingredient amounts and dosage vary and occasionally other ingredients were added. See also "Discussion of Influenza," *Proceedings of the Royal Society of Medicine: General Reports*, 12 (1919): 57; *The Lancet*, 2 (Nov. 23, 1919): 695-97; *British Medical Journal*, 2 (July 27, 1918): 91.

[20]Ministry of Health, *Report on the Pandemic*, 475-76.

[21]Manchester, *1918 Report*, 34; *Ibid.*, for 1919, 181-Table 2; *Manchester Guardian*, Dec. 5, 1918.

[22]Manchester, *1918 Report*, 66; *Ibid.*, for 1919, 179.

particularly severe cases.[23] Finally, on March 18, 1919, a ward was opened in Monsall Hospital for influenza cases complicated by pneumonia.[24]

Sudden onset was a frightening and difficult problem. "At one school," Niven reported, "I observed the children falling ill. They simply dropped on their desk like a plant whose roots have been poisoned. . . ."[25] Tales of people collapsing at work or even in the street are common. Medical help was difficult to get throughout the period. Many doctors were away in the service--the Manchester Medical Society reported membership of 403 in 1918 and 455 in 1919 but so many were away that in 1916 emergency efforts were required to keep the Society's library open--and just getting to see a doctor was not easy.[26] The Manchester War Medical Committee sought the release of doctors from the colors, especially after the armistice, arguing that local physicians were on the verge of collapse from working around the clock. Pressure to get doctors returned from military service had limited success.[27]

Although a variety of treatments--some quite bizarre, such as intravenous infusions of oil of garlic--were prescribed, Manchester's doctors, like those of the rest of the country, favored alcohol, usually whiskey, although brandy was not uncommon. To the outrage of the populace, though perhaps to their better health, the supply of whiskey was controlled by the government to ensure that supplies of grain would be used for food. Although some doctors insisted that alcohol was of no value, the popular feeling was that the authorities "could be said to have murdered men and women through this shortage of whiskey." Public protests were organized.[28]

---

[23] *Ibid.*, 105; (Manchester) *Evening Chronicle*, Feb. 20, 1919.

[24] Ministry of Health, *Report on the Pandemic*, 475.

[25] *Ibid.*, 472.

[26] Annual Reports of the Manchester Medical Society for 1915-1918, 10; *Ibid.* for 1919, 10, Central Lib. See also John V. Pickstone, *Medicine and Industrial Society: A History of Hospital Development in Manchester and its Region, 1752-1946* (Manchester, 1985), 206.

[27] (Manchester) *Evening Chronicle*, March 10, 1919.

[28] *Ibid.*, March 5 (Quotation), March 10, 1919.

In the end, disgust was the attitude toward the entire health profession as expressed by a letter in the *Guardian*:

> On March 1 you published a letter written by an eminent physician in which he very strongly recommended the use of solution of permanganate of potash for influenza. On February 28, at the Medical Conference on Hygiene, sitting in London, the chairman, another eminent physician stated that the use of such a solution was a 'horrible remedy.' Which of the two is to be believed? The other day I was talking to a district nurse in a suburb only a short distance from Manchester, and was told that she was attending patients prescribed by four medical men, yet each doctor had a different method of dealing with this plague. It is more than likely that such differences obtain all over the country. Why do not the medical men in Manchester and district have a meeting, decide what is actually required, and have their decision put before the proper authorities?[29]

An estimate of the economic impact of the pandemic is difficult to make. The economic disruption of the war, with labor shortages and heroic measures to ensure adequate production of necessary items and acceptance of shortages in other areas, clouds the picture of production curves. Some measure can be gotten however, by looking at absenteeism at businesses and factories for which such records are available. Based on the Ministry of Health's block survey after the fact, Manchester had well over 100,000 cases in the first wave alone. On July 8, 1918, Messers. Lewis reported 15% of their workers away from their jobs. A month later, the local artillery shell factory noted that 22.68% of its workers had been out with flu and Armstrong and Witworth's had lost 20.78%. The Crossley Brothers plant indicated that "at the height of the epidemic" 16.85% of its workers were absent.[30] These rates may be compared with the report of the Medical Officer of Health concerning the pandemic of the early 1890s that a survey of 146 establishments with some 32,000 workers showed only about 2% away from work due to influenza.[31]

[29]*Manchester Guardian*, March 11, 1919.

[30]Ministry of Health, *Report on the Pandemic*, 473.

[31]Tatham, 61.

It is undeniable that some people used the pandemic as an excuse to stay home, but the Medical Officer of Health and private physicians repeatedly advised ten days to three weeks rest depending on the severity of the attack. The danger of relapse, which was more likely to develop into pneumonia, was emphasized as part of the importance of resting until truly well, and according to Niven, "employers. . . should recognize the importance of this precaution."[32] While such advice was clearly in the best interest of the victim, it certainly increased the cost to employers. Although conversion to a cash approximation is almost impossible--the limited samples available even make it difficult to figure total days lost since those samples fail to provide evidence concerning the average length of sick leave--the cost was clearly enormous.

Contemporary public health was unable to prevent the deadly and expensive impact of the pandemic. Manchester, lucky to have an MOH like Niven, who saw the virtue of centralized health activity, still suffered on a scale comparable to the rest of the country. Public aid with food, fuel, and nursing was of much more value than treatment by local physicians, but in reality Mancunians in 1918-19 were little better off in the face of the epidemic than their ancestors had been in the face of cholera in 1832. Their expressions of frustration and fear, even refusing to go to the aid of suffering friends and relatives, were much like those of people in the 1980s facing A.I.D.S.

---

[32] *Manchester Guardian*, June 25, June 26, 1918.

Chapter 6: Atlanta

Francine King

Atlanta, founded in 1837, had only a population of about 12,000 when it was devastated in 1864. Its growth, like that of other Southern cities, was slow during the latter part of the 19th century, but by 1900 its population was approaching 90,000 and it "had become a regional metropolis. . . ."[1] Over the next two decades it grew more dramatically, becoming a Southeastern business center and prominent nationally in the textile industry.[2] In 1909 the city hosted the South's first national automobile show, and although slowed by economic problems and the lack of good roads in the region, the automotive industry became an important element in the city's early 20th century growth. Autos were generating forty to fifty million dollars a year in business for Atlanta by 1917. While, for the time, cars remained possessions of the wealthy, Atlanta also had a streetcar system that provided the everyday citizen with transportation. This system with 51,500 miles of track in 1912 compared quite favorably with other provincial U.S. cities such as Denver, Salt Lake City, and Albany.[3] Atlanta's emergence as a business and

---

[1]Truman A. Hartshorn, *et al.*, *Metropolis in Georgia: Atlanta's Rise as a Major Transaction Center* (Cambridge, 1976), 3.

[2]*Ibid.*; Howard L. Preston, *Automobile Age Atlanta: The Making of a Southern Metropolis, 1900-1935* (Athens, GA, 1979), 1-2.

[3]*Ibid.*, 17, 37, 49-50.

commercial center in the first decades of the century was highlighted by the $25,000,000 sale of the Coca Cola Company in 1919.[4]

Although he died in 1889, Henry Grady, prominent editor of the *Atlanta Constitution* would have welcomed the city's development. Grady had been instrumental in encouraging Atlantans to become a part of the New South. He had promulgated a new image for the region: that of a powerful and prosperous industrialized region.[5] The city, if not the South, was beginning to live up to the dream. In addition to the commercial growth noted, Atlanta was becoming well known as a convention center. It had secured the Sixth District Federal Reserve Bank and Fort Gordon, an army cantonment, that served as a replacement camp during World War I. The federal government was spending approximately $25,000,000 annually in the area. Another stimulus to Atlanta's economic growth was the Southeastern Fair Association, formed by the Chamber of Commerce in 1915 to promote Atlanta's business interests. This association leased the site of Lakewood and sponsored annual fairs and scheduled popular summer events.[6]

Grady left another heritage--boosterism--that sometimes caused Atlanta's governmental and commercial leaders to downplay problems such as the danger of yellow fever in 1905 and influenza in 1918. Sometimes called "the Atlanta Spirit," this attitude verged on the hysterical. Convinced that ". . . economic prosperity depended on maintaining Atlanta's reputation for salubrity. . . .,[7] the city fathers sought to keep health problems from becoming known. The Chamber of Commerce ". . . argued that Atlanta's position as the region's leading city required it to be come the examplar of

---

[4]Franklin M. Garrett, *Atlanta and Environs: A Chronicle of Its People and Events* (Athens, GA, 1969), II: 767-68.

[5]E. Merton Coulter, *Georgia: A Short History* (Chapel Hill, NC, 1973), 383-84.

[6]Workers of the Writers' Program of the W.P.A. in the State of Georgia, *Atlanta: A City of the Modern South* (Michigan, 1973), 194-95.

[7]Stuart Galishoff, "Germs Know No Color Line: Black Health and Public Policy in Atlanta, 1900-1918," *Journal of the History of Medicine and Allied Sciences*, 40 (Jan., 1985): 32.

Southern cities in sanitation and public health."[8] This attitude was carried so far that water and sewer services were extended into black sections, which before and after got little in the way of city services. This unusual concern for the black population was due to fear that epidemics in that group would tarnish the city's reputation.[9] Thus the pattern of concern about and sometimes hiding health problems was established well before 1918.

Growth had not come without problems and social stress, however. A race riot in 1906 followed by some of the strictest segregation codes in the country, a major city fire in 1917 exacerbating a housing shortage in the city, a war-fueled burgeoning of the cost of living (in 1917 coal, the primary home heating fuel, was put on a cash in advance basis) all suggested that the city had problems to solve in the second decade of the twentieth century.[10] The Atlanta Spirit was unbowed, however, and it would continue to be so in the face of influenza, although even the doggedly sanguine *Official History of Fulton County* acknowledged that the epidemic was "the worst ever known, and heroic measures had to be taken to check the spread of the disease."[11]

The state of Georgia had 30,768 reported cases of influenza in 1918, and undoubtedly very many unreported ones--either mild or simply unattended by health care professionals.[12] Atlanta was quite lucky, however, for it did not see the typical wave pattern of the epidemic. The summer wave went almost completely unnoticed, with no press comment even when it caused problems on the Western Front. Generally the least deadly, the first wave kept its victims off their feet for no more than a week. Any cases in Atlanta were simply ignored. Atlanta also got off easily in the third wave that occurred most places in February-March of 1919. There was a renewal

---

[8]John Ellis and Stuart Galishoff, "Atlanta's Water Supply, 1865-1918," *Maryland Historian*, 8 (Spring, 1977): 17.

[9]*Ibid.*, 19.

[10]Hartshorn, 44; Garrett, II: 737.

[11]Walter G. Cooper, *The Official History of Fulton County* (Spartanburg, SC, 1978), 382.

[12]"Morbidity Report of Georgia, 1918," *Annual Report of Georgia State Board of Health*, 1918, 53.

of the infection in the Atlanta area in mid-January, 1919, causing some problems in schools in small towns outside the city,[13] but compared to the third wave in many places this was minimal. Atlanta really had to cope only with the second wave, the most deadly.

Unfortunately extant records make it difficult to be very precise about the numbers of Atlantans struck by the disease. City Health Department records have been lost and no 1918 Atlanta report was filed with the State Health Department. Tax supported Grady Memorial Hospital's records are available. However, early in the epidemic twelve nurses fell ill, and since a shortage of doctors and nurses already existed due to the war effort, officials immediately closed the hospital to all influenza patients and required all the medical staff to wear "flu masks."[14] Those records--even admissions records--therefore offer little help to those interested in the impact of influenza. Information must come from the newspapers, and they tended to follow the generally upbeat line taken by the city's booster-oriented officials i.e. Atlanta does not have a problem. Popular memory differed, however: "They were dying just like leaves off of them trees. . . .," one citizen remembered.[15]

In newspaper comments, Dr. J. P. Kennedy, Atlanta City Health Officer, consistently reported improving health conditions and low death rates.[16] According to these articles, the total number of influenza cases reported was approximately 3,000. Between October 2nd and 17th, 2,000 cases were reported. On October 18, a total of 2,500 cases had been reported.[17] It seems almost incredible that 83% of the total cases would occur in sixteen days and 20% of those overnight.[18] Kennedy's statistics must

---

[13]*The Atlanta Semi-Weekly Journal*, Jan. 14, 1919.

[14]*Atlanta Journal*, Oct. 9, 1918; *Atlanta Constitution*, Oct. 10, 1918.

[15]Clifford M. Kuhn, Harlon E. Joye, and E. Bernard West, *Living Atlanta: An Oral History of the City, 1914-1948* (Athens, GA and London, 1990), 28.

[16]*The Atlanta Georgian*, Oct. 18, 1918, First edition.

[17]*Atlanta Journal*, Oct. 18, 20, 1918.

[18]*The Atlanta Georgian*, Oct. 22, 1918, First edition.

be regarded as questionable and almost certainly substantially low. If he is accurate, in fact, Fort Gordon soldiers had as many cases (see below) as the entire civilian population of the city.

A general analysis by Kennedy for the week of October 21 gives the morbidity and mortality of the city. He reported 81 deaths for the week--53 whites and 28 blacks. The majority of the fatalities were between ages of 30 and 40, and the second largest group consisted of those between 40 and 50. The death rate was approximately 30 per 1,000 cases. Thus a conservative estimate indicates that, in a four week period, Atlanta experienced 320 deaths. Blacks, who made up 33.45% of the city population, were 34.57% of the deaths. This does not suggest a disporprotionate impact in the black community, and the black press did not suggest that its constituency was suffering more than the rest of the community. Its coverage was quite similar to that of the white press.

The first influenza cases reported in the Atlanta area were at Fort Gordon, to the southwest of the city.[19] During the week of October 2, ten deaths were reported and 138 soldiers were hospitalized there. The total number of cases at the camp had risen to 2,941 by the second week in October.[20] The Atlanta Red Cross and the Georgia Terrace, a women's social auxiliary, made 100,000 gauze flu masks for the soldiers.[21] As a result, all soldiers were required to wear the masks to avoid spreading the virus any further. Roads at the camp were oiled with an antiseptic that supposedly "kept down" the disease germs that travel in the dust and air.[22] Soldiers were not allowed into the Atlanta city limits and the Masons' Association of Fulton County cancelled its weekly dances and entertainment events for

---

[19] *Atlanta Constitution*, Oct. 2, 1918. During the autumn of the year, 19,429 deaths were reported among American troops. Fort Gordon's experience was part of a larger national phenomena which led to the theory that the Spanish influenza infection was rooted in the armed forces.

[20] *The Atlanta Georgian*, Oct. 8, 1918, Home edition.

[21] *Ibid.*, Oct. 5, 1918.

[22] *Ibid.*, Oct. 4, 1918.

military men.[23] Another precautionary measure taken required soldiers to sleep outdoors rather in barracks. Nonetheless, deaths were a daily occurrence. It was reported that coffins were "stacked like cordwood" awaiting return to the families of the deceased young men.[24] Landlords attempted to oust families of soldiers stationed at the army camp; however, the Atlanta Chamber of Commerce Housing Department interceded in these actions. City ordinances restricted landlords' options to imposing quarantines on infected dwellings.[25]

Although the disease was severe at Fort Gordon, Dr. Kennedy reported on October 4 only five deaths from influenza and emphasized that Atlanta registered the lowest death rate in a year. The city, in his opinion, was virtually free of the disease. Kennedy further asserted that the five deaths were in the "colored section" and were caused by neglect.[26] On October 7 in an action suggesting that Kennedy's optimism might just be the Atlanta Spirit at work, the General Council of the City of Atlanta passed an ordinance stating:

> From after the approval of this ordinance, each and all schools, churches, theaters, moving picture shows of all kinds, vaudeville, dance halls, pool and billiard rooms shall close and remain closed for and during the next two months, or until such time as this ordinance shall be amended or repealed prior to two months period, however, that if the epidemic of influenza continues at the end of two months period this Council will pass an additional ordinance continuing the closing of the named places to some future time to be named. All street cars, buses or similar modes of public conveyance shall operate with the windows open except during rain.[27]

---

[23]*Ibid.*, Oct. 5, 1918.

[24]*Ibid.*, Oct. 8, 1918; Franklin M. Garrett, interview with author, Atlanta, GA, Sept. 5, 1988; Garrett, II: 735.

[25]*Atlanta Constitution*, Oct. 9, 1918.

[26]*The Atlanta Georgian*, Oct. 14, 1918, First edition.

[27]City of Atlanta, Minutes of the General Council, Oct. 7, 1918, 373.

After passage of the ordinance, the Health Department reaffirmed its view that an epidemic did not exist in Atlanta, and that the city's schools and theaters had been closed only as a precautionary measure.[28] Nonetheless, Kennedy conceded that "the plague" was on the increase and the disease was serious. He estimated that each doctor in Atlanta was treating fifteen to twenty flu patients a week.[29] The city's major newspaper supported the official line by continuing to present a non-crisis situation to the public. Although not in a panic, another paper seemed more concerned and referred to influenza as "a great and terrifying menace to the public health. . . ."[30]

On October 8, the Health Department announced several seemingly contradictory policies. First, it was stated that violations of the public gathering ordinances would carry a fine of two hundred dollars for each occurrence. Second, the ordinances were declared not to cover the upcoming Southeastern fair, and officials hoped that the influenza conditions in the city would not cause the closing of businesses.[31] Third, all physicians were asked to report cases and reminded that they would be in violation of federal regulations if they failed to heed the request.[32] It sounds almost as if the Health Department prepared its recommendations in conjunction with the Chamber of Commerce.

Atlanta city officials proposed several preventive measures to help curb the epidemic. City welfare nurses were required to visit all victims of the flu to assess the extent of the illness and to provide medical advice. Factory workers, shop employees and downtown shoppers were required to wear face masks.[33] Police were expected to prevent citizens from "expectorating in the streets," and garbage removal and street sweeping were

---

[28] *Atlanta Constitution*, Oct. 10, 1918.

[29] *The Atlanta Georgian*, Oct. 8, 1918, Home edition.

[30] *The Atlanta Semi-Weekly Journal*, Oct. 15, 1918.

[31] *The Atlanta Georgian*, Oct. 8, 1918, Home edition; *Atlanta Constitution*, Oct. 8, 1918.

[32] *Ibid.*, Oct. 12, 1918.

[33] *Ibid.*, Oct. 10, 1918.

prohibited during the hours when large numbers of Atlantans were in the downtown area.[34] These actions, taken by a city which officially denied that it was faced with an epidemic, parallel those taken in cities that made no bones about having a very serious one indeed.

City officials and institutions took immediate steps to enforce preventive ordinances and take precautions against the spread of the disease. Crowded street cars were an obvious problem. In 1918 they carried 85,481,204 passengers. J. C. Miliner, a cotton grinder, was arrested for closing a car window, and his protests that he thought the public had been requested rather than ordered to keep the windows open were ignored.[35] As previously noted, Grady Hospital decided to protect its staff and patients with other ills by rejecting flu victims. Daily announcements of closings and cancellations of public events were publicized in the newspapers, and the criminal and civil court systems closed operations for thirty days.[36]

Influenza prevention touched every phase of daily life. Dr. Claude Smith, city bacteriologist, suggested that offices should eliminate common drinking cups, which increased the spread of the disease. Another doctor suggested that sulfur be placed in the bottom of each shoe to ward off the disease.[37] A choirmaster suggested that citizens speak the vowel "ah" like singers to allow spray to reach all parts of the throat for complete destruction of germs. Mrs. Hunnicut, a fashion-conscious citizen, suggested that women wear veils rather than "flu masks" since they were stylish and much more becoming.[38] Commercial advertisement of flu prevention products

---

[34] *Ibid.*

[35] *The Atlanta Georgian*, Oct. 15, 1918, Final edition; Preston, 48-Table 3.1.

[36] *Atlanta Constitution*, Oct. 10, 1918; *Atlanta Journal*, Oct. 8, 1918; *The Atlanta Independent*, Oct. 12, Nov. 2, 1918.

[37] *Atlanta Constitution*, Oct. 12, 1918.

[38] *Ibid.*, Oct. 9, 1918.

flourished, promoting nose douches, gargling with Listerine-Dioxagen, massaging with Eucalyptic salve and other such quack nostrums.[39]

A positive attitude was also proposed as a preventive measure. Dr. Wood Hutchinson suggested that an individual should not worry seriously about the disease because, in his estimation, chances of contracting the influenza were only 1 in 150. He further estimated that an individual's chances of dying if infected were approximately 1 in 20. Knowledge and a positive attitude could prevent fear, Dr. Hutchinson wrote, and individuals could thereby prevent being infected by the virus.[40]

Either a smile was no preventive or Atlantans were glum, for the influenza epidemic caused a severe labor shortage throughout the city. So many employees in the Atlanta area were reported ill from influenza that several companies were forced to curtail their services. A Southern Bell Telephone manager reported up to 600 operators absent from work during the peak of the epidemic. The company requested that the public not make any calls, social or business, "unless absolutely necessary."[41] Clearing House Banks, which collected most out-of-town tourists' checks, notified the public of reduced hours of business because so many bank employees were confined to their homes with influenza. Banking officials requested that customers make deposits "before one o'clock except on Saturday," when deposits were accepted only before eleven o'clock.[42] Cancellations of conventions were also a concern. Fred Houser, Secretary of Atlanta's Convention Bureau, feared that the influenza epidemic might cause a downward trend in the convention business, for several of the year's 129 gatherings had already been cancelled.[43]

---

[39]*Ibid.*; Similar notes run in every issue of *The Atlanta Semi-Weekly Journal* from Oct. 18, 1919 into March of 1919 and in *The Atlanta Independent* from Oct. 19, 1918 into March of 1919.

[40]*Sunday American* (*The Atlanta Georgian*), Oct. 13, 1918.

[41]*Atlanta Constitution*, Oct. 11, 1918.

[42]*Ibid.*

[43]*Ibid.*, Oct. 9, 1918.

One special event was conspicuously exempt from cancellation, however: the Southeastern Fair. Held every October, the fair was Atlanta's largest annual event, attracting more visitors from over the entire Southeast than any other Atlanta enterprise. In three buildings, exhibits of farm products, machinery, canned foods, and handicrafts were shown. Food and drink, games, and traveling shows provided a carnival atmosphere. The display of livestock and poultry was the most significant in the South.[44] Since the Chamber of Commerce owned 100% of the common stock of the Southeastern Fair, the organization did not allow it to close. To do so would be to admit of problems that the Atlanta Spirit could not overcome.

On October 10, the Atlanta Advertising Club held a luncheon at which H. G. Hasting, President of the Southeastern Fair Association; R. M. Stublin, Secretary and General Manager; Dillard Jackson, Chairman of the Educational Committee; and Fred Houser, Secretary of the Atlanta Convention Bureau,[45] discussed the value of the fair to Atlanta. On October 12, newspaper headlines encouraged the public to attend the fair, noting that the Public Board of Health had declared the fair a safe environment.[46] The three major newspapers reported several thousand Atlantans attending the fair despite the city's nervousness over the virus.[47] Dr. T. F. Abercrombie, Secretary of the State Health Department, allowed the fair to remain open despite of a telegram "to all State Health Authorities" from United States Surgeon General Rupert Blue, who advised "discontinuing all public meetings, closing all schools and places of public amusement as done in other states on appearance of local outbreaks."[48] Dr. Abercrombie and City of Atlanta Health Officer Dr. J. P. Kennedy did visit and inspect the fair. Both

---

[44]"Convention to be Held," *The City Builder*, (Oct., 1918), 26; *Atlanta Constitution*, Oct. 9, 1918.

[45]*Atlanta Journal*, Oct. 10, 1918.

[46]*Atlanta Constitution*, Oct. 12, 1918.

[47]*The Atlanta Georgian*, Oct. 15, 1918, First edition.

[48]Minutes of the Georgia State Board of Health, Oct. 18, 1918, 347.

men approved of health conditions and did not recommend any changes.[49] In spite of the visitation, however, Dr. Abercrombie called a Health Board meeting on October 17 to consider closing the fair. (At this point in the progression of the virus, Atlanta had officially reported only 2,500 cases and 81 deaths from the disease. The Board's concern suggests the problem was much greater than the official statistics suggest.) In the end, the Board compromised by allowing the fair to remain open but requiring that everyone who entered must wear a "flu mask."[50]

Public protest erupted over the decision to allow the fair to open. Atlanta's Theater Managers Association was indignant over the city officials' decision to allow the public to view shows in enclosed tents at the fair while prohibiting the viewing of shows in ventilated theaters. The issue was taken to the Safety Committee of the Chamber of Commerce, which decided to investigate but ultimately declined to adopt a resolution reopening theaters.[51] Edgar A. Neely, a theater manager, contended that not only were Atlanta's theater owners being "deprived of a means of livelihood, but also closing of theaters was harmful to the liberty bond drive." (Liberty bond sales were promoted in theater presentations.) He believed that the fair was instrumental in spreading the flu and causing a longer period of quarantine.[52]

The Reverend R. M. Lipham, pastor of the Calvary Methodist Church, spoke out for the Atlanta church community. He asserted that the fair would spread the disease more rapidly than would a well ventilated church, and he wanted officials to put the churches on "equal footing with the fair."[53] In spite of local dissent, however, the Southeastern Fair remained open, and the theaters, churches, and schools remained closed--a testimony to the clout of the Chamber of Commerce.

---

[49]*The Atlanta Georgian*, Oct. 16, 1918, Home edition; "Statement by the Health Officers," *The City Builder* (Nov., 1918), 22.

[50]*The Atlanta Georgian*, Oct. 19, 1918, First edition.

[51]*Ibid.*, Oct. 15, 1918, Afternoon edition.

[52]*Ibid.*, Oct. 16, 1918, Home edition.

[53]*Ibid.*, Oct. 18, 1918, First edition.

Despite the severity of the epidemic, the Southeastern Fair was heralded as a huge success, and only a few Atlantans stayed away. Participation and attendance incentives were offered by fair officials and businessmen. Merchants gave employees a holiday to attend the fair and crowds were drawn to the fair by special admission on "School Day." The *Atlanta Independent*, with a predominantly black readership, made a point of urging that children take advantage of the ten cents admission on School Day, without any mention of the danger of infection.[54] Governor and Mrs. Dorsey attended the fair and drew a crowd of 25,000.[55] Fair officials reported that over one million individuals from all over the Southeast attended the event. The crowds were recorded as the largest in the fair's history. Amusement tents were packed to capacity.[56] Apparently fair goers were not intimidated by concern about illness, or perhaps the official effort to downplay the presence of an epidemic was effective.

Other businesses, however, did experience a decline. Trade was hindered by the disease combined with orders from the federal government to curtail the use of electric power. Banking clearings for the peak period of the epidemic in October reflected a decrease in money-making transactions in the city of Atlanta. Bankers indicated an interruption in many lines of trade due to closings of places of business due to the influenza and to the reduction of power. One report cited a weekly statement of the Atlanta Clearing House Association which placed clearings through local national banks at $6,000,000 less than the previous week, due to economic conditions attributed to the epidemic. The report added that, "with the influenza ban lifted, business here next week will again hum with activity, despite the power conservation."[57] The cotton market also exhibited a marked decline during

---

[54]*Atlanta Journal*, Oct. 5, 1918; *The Atlanta Georgian*, Oct. 16, 1918, Evening edition; *The Atlanta Independent*, Sept. 28, 1918.

[55]*The Atlanta Georgian*, Oct. 18, 1918, First edition.

[56]*Sunday American* (*The Atlanta Georgian*), Oct. 20, 1918.

[57]*Ibid.*, Oct. 27, 1918.

the epidemic. A statement issued on October 28 shows a downward trend in cotton shipments, stocks, and sales for the previous week.[58]

Atlanta city officials were instrumental in ensuring that the city suffered only minimal economic deterioration. They made heroic efforts to convince citizens that a serious influenza epidemic did not exist within the city limits. Dr. Kennedy, City Health Officer, proposed, on October 22, to lift the ban on public gatherings and reported a stabilizing situation of 36 deaths from Saturday to Tuesday.[59] A heated debate took place in a special session of the City Council on October 25 when Mayor Candler, theater managers and Dr. Kennedy fought to repeal the closing ordinances of October 7. The Atlanta Board of Health staff opposed Dr. Kennedy because the Board staff felt the epidemic remained serious. The City Council, however, overruled the Board and lifted the ban, showing once again that the concern in city government was more with profit and image than health.[60]

The City Council recommended that schools reopen on November 4, unless the Health Board made other recommendations. The situation was reported to have further stabilized; only 14 deaths had been reported in a twenty-four hour period.[61] Thus, in the opinion of "city fathers," the serious influenza condition of 1918 was officially terminated.

The Spanish influenza pandemic of 1918 struck the population of Atlanta a violent blow but resulted in few humanitarian gestures on the part of the city fathers. City officials and the Chamber of Commerce tended to deny that the epidemic existed, and were inclined against preventive measures that might interfere with major business activities. The "Atlanta Spirit" was at work. The official statistics are incredible. If correct, then 20% of the total cases in Atlanta occurred among telephone operators, a group not particularly known for undue susceptibility to influenza. Although

---

[58]*The Atlanta Georgian*, Oct. 28, 1918, First edition.

[59]City of Atlanta, Minutes of General Council, Oct. 25, 1918, 386; *The Atlanta Georgian*, Oct. 26, 1918, First edition.

[60]*Ibid.*

[61]*Atlanta Journal* Oct. 25, 1918.

Atlanta lost many its young and productive citizens, neither the downtown business district nor the Southeastern Fair closed even during the peak of the epidemic. A December 16 resolution to increase the funding of the Contagious Disease Hospital was the only significant concession the town leaders made to the epidemic. City officials had played a dangerous game with the health of the city, and they were lucky enough that Atlanta had a relatively limited outbreak of the epidemic. It was a triumph of the "Atlanta Spirit."

Chapter 7: Chicago

Paul A. Buelow

The Spanish flu of 1918 and 1919 provides a revealing light in which to view a large city's actions during a crisis. An examination of the words and actions of the city's public health officials, hospitals, charitable organizations, and the public itself during the Spanish flu may facilitate a greater understanding of the ways in which society responded to an epidemic of life-threatening disease.

One of the basic challenges involved in public health is balancing proper preparedness with over-publicizing a threat, which might lead to ill-advised action. Certainly the government and the business community desire calm and oppose measures which could be seen as leading to panic or a business slow-down. The Chicago Department of Health in its weekly *Bulletin* for August 31, 1918, stated that in the past, when no one knew what caused disease, cities actually tried to conceal from the public the extent or virulence of an epidemic. In a typically Progressive vein, the *Bulletin* said now that health officers know something about causes and prevention, "publicity and education [are]. . . the most important factors in public health protection."[1] The *Bulletin* carried the heading, "Sanitary Instruction Is Even More Important than Sanitary Legislation." But properly publicizing a threat

---

[1]*Bulletin*, Chicago School of Sanitary Instruction 12 (August 31, 1918): 157. I would like to thank Professors Burton Bledstein and Perry Duis of the University of Illinois at Chicago, who provided initial guidance and pointed out resources in the preparation of the thesis from which this chapter is excerpted.

to the public's health proves to be a delicate task, and when officials suggest closing businesses, they find themselves between conflicting interests.[2] The reactions of Chicago's health officials to the epidemic illustrate this conflict.

In late 1918, apart from its preoccupation with the war, Chicago was busy. It was dealing with immigrants from overseas as well as migrating workers from the South. Its population had swelled to almost 2.6 million, almost exactly half of New York's size, but nearly a million more than the third-largest U.S. city, Philadelphia. Housing was a problem, and overcrowding in low-income districts was common. William Hale "Big Bill" Thompson was mayor, and politics was a big part of city life.

Chicago newspapers were headlining war news: "Advance on St. Quentin," "Class Hatred Rules Russia; Human Life Valueless," and "Twenty Years in Prison for Draft Evaders." Writers detailed President Wilson's announcement of the fourth Liberty Loan Drive; Chicago's goal was set at $250 million.[3] Sports news focused on the World Series (Boston's Red Sox defeated Chicago's Cubs in four straight) and on another event--the forthcoming National Amateur Athletic Association track and field meet, to be held from Friday to Sunday, September 20 to 22, at the Great Lakes Naval Station, about 32 miles north of the city on Lake Michigan. Athletes from all over the country were to compete.

It was at the Great Lakes Station that the first Chicago-area case of Spanish flu was recorded, on Sunday, September 8. By that date the epidemic had been spreading in East Coast states for almost two weeks, but Chicago papers did not take notice of this Midwestern outbreak for over a week. The flu was first featured as a news story on Monday, September 16, though not on the front page. The article told of the situation at the Great Lakes Station.[4] Precautionary measures were to be taken. The 50,000 men stationed there in preparation for advance to Europe were to be treated daily

---

[2]See Bradford Luckingham, *Epidemic in the Southwest, 1918-1919* (El Paso, 1984), 13, 25, 26; and Charles E. Rosenberg, *The Cholera Years: America in 1832, 1849, and 1866* (Chicago, 1966), 19-30.

[3]*Chicago Daily News*, Sept. 9, 1918.

[4]*Chicago Tribune*, Sept. 16, 1918.

with nose and throat sprays, and "sneeze screens" were to be set up in sleeping quarters. Navy surgeon Dr. Owen J. Mink warned the men not to wear damp clothing, and Captain William A. Moffett, the Station Commander, suspended indoor work as much as possible so as to get the "Jackies" (short for "Blue-Jacket") outside into the healthful outdoor air. But the problem at Great Lakes was not very serious. The writer said, "Only a few. . . have been affected."

The danger of contagion soon became obvious, however. After the 16th of September, Chicago newspapers carried accounts of the Spanish flu every day until nearly the end of October. Officials at Great Lakes had closed parts of the camp, and on the 17th, a front-page story in the *Tribune* carried the headline, "Epidemic of Influenza Quarantines 4,000 Jackies." Towns on the north shore were already experiencing the realities of the epidemic. On September 9, the day after the first occurrence at Great Lakes, Winnetka had its first reported case. The flu virus was to follow a roughly north-to-south route around and through the Chicago metropolitan area, hitting the southern areas as much as four weeks after it appeared in the north.

Table 7.1

Influenza Mortality by Age, October, 1918 Disease

Disease	*Age at Death (in Years)*								
	0-1	1-10	10-20	20-30	30-40	40-50	50-60	60-70	70-90
Pneumonia	172	555	174	737	651	227	113	57	59
Influenza	174	793	312	1356	1124	343	145	88	39
Total	346	1348	486	2093	1775	570	258	145	98

Source: John Dill Robertson, *A Report on An Epidemic of Influenza in the City of Chicago in the Fall of 1918.* Reprinted from the Octennial Report, 1911-18, Education Series No. 15 (Chicago, 1918), 31--Table 8.

In contrast to previous influenza epidemics, the Spanish flu was much more productive of fatal complications, such as pneumonia, and consequently much more deadly. Ordinary influenza was fatal to the very young and very old, but this disease was far more so in a different age group: young adults, aged 20 to 40, the ages of parents with young children.[5] In Chicago, this unusual mortality was quite pronounced. See Table 7.1. Table 7.2 provides data on relative increases in mortality from both influenza and pneumonia in Chicago. The much greater increases in people aged 20-30 (13,800%) and 30-40 (21,090%) contrast strikingly with the 5-10 (13,950%) and 10-15 (10,950%) age groups. By comparison, the increase in mortality of those under 5 during the first month of the 1890-92 influenza epidemic in Chicago was 73.6%, with 110.1% for the 20-30 year-olds, and 154.3% for the 30-40 year-olds.[6]

Table 7.2

Relative Increases in Mortality by Age,
Sept. 22 to Nov. 12, 1918,

0-5	5-10	10-20	20-30	30-40	40-50	50-60	Over 60
2545%	13950%	10950%	30800%	21090%	3910%	2242%	1370%

Source: John Dill Robertson, *A Report on An Epidemic of Influenza in the City of Chicago in the Fall of 1918.* Reprinted from the Octennial Report, 1911-18, Education Series No. 15 (Chicago, 1918), 34--Chart 16.

The Chicago Department of Health had used the city's daily, weekly, and monthly publications, including foreign language dailies, to discuss prevention and treatment of various diseases. Other means of publicizing the threat of communicable disease were used as well, among them notices posted in street cars and elevated trains warning against the danger of spitting, coughing, and sneezing in public. The notices were part of a program that had been planned and implemented before the flu epidemic became a concern, but proved quite applicable. The copy from one such notice ran:[7]

---

[5]John Dill Robertson, *A Report on An Epidemic of Influenza in the City of Chicago in the Fall of 1918.* Reprinted from the Octennial Report, 1911-1918, Education Series No. 15 (Chicago, 1918), 32-34. See also Gerald F. Pyle, *The Diffusion of Influenza: Patterns and Paradigms* (Totowa, NJ, 1986), 40.

[6]Robertson, 38--Chart 18.

[7]Robertson, 54-55.

> SNEEZING, COUGHING, SPITTING IN PUBLIC PLACES HELP TO SPREAD SUCH DANGEROUS DISEASES AS INFLUENZA, PNEUMONIA, DIPHTHERIA, AND CONSUMPTION. IN 1917 THE GERMS THAT CAUSE THESE FOUR DISEASES KILLED 10,220 PEOPLE IN CHICAGO. COVER YOUR MOUTH AND NOSE WHEN YOU SNEEZE OR COUGH AND HELP TO KEEP CHICAGO HEALTHY.

The *Tribune* story of Tuesday, September 17, reporting that a quarantine had been set up at Great Lakes, stated that "several hundred" cases had occurred, and that "All buildings available, including the Y.M.C.A. quarters, are being used for the sick men." On Wednesday the same paper headlined the story of the flu in the nation's military camps (called "cantonments"): "In 3 Army Camps U.S. Finds Spanish Influenza Peril." Also on the first page were stories telling of seventy dead in New England and official action making the flu a reportable disease in New York state. The paper also related that the first marriage in quarantine had been performed at Great Lakes. Immediately after the ceremony the groom had to hurry back to his barracks, to remain there at least five more days![8] The flu had indeed gained news value.

The National A.A.A. games were still on the schedule at the Naval Training Station, despite the worsening health situation there. Newspaper stories on the 18th and 19th told of 300 athletes from all over the country who would be competing. Officials expected 75,000 spectators to be on hand to watch events that were to rival the Olympics. Other stories noted that Army cantonments around the country had already had over 20,000 cases of Spanish flu. Fort Sheridan had 120 cases more than the day before, and North Shore towns like Glencoe and Winnetka were closing schools and theaters. Soldiers from the Home Guard in these communities padlocked saloons and patrolled closed school-yards, and local Boy Scout troops distributed daily bulletins about the epidemic.[9]

---

[8] *Chicago Tribune*, Sept. 18, 1918.

[9] A. A. Hoehling, *The Great Epidemic* (Boston, 1961). 44.

As though to demonstrate the explosive dissemination of this disease, by September 19th the quarantine at Great Lakes had been expanded to include over 1,000 men. Health Commissioner Dr. John Dill Robertson released a statement to the effect that it now seemed likely the epidemic of Spanish flu would spread to the city proper. He added, though, that with proper care and precautions citizens could minimize its effects. The greatest danger, he said, was from pneumonia resulting from a case of flu. The press release described typical flu symptoms and advised a treatment of bed rest, free movement of the bowels (an important part of therapeutics at the time), and a light diet. People were to be wary of "droplet infection," from sneezers and coughers.[10] A cluster of flu-related stories, including Robertson's warnings, was headlined "Grip Epidemic at Great Lakes Under Control."[11] This headline, and Dr. Robertson's low-key approach to warning the populace of the city, are curious. In a few days the number of cases at the Naval Station would increase tremendously. Judging from reports coming from other parts of the country at the time, especially the East Coast, this could have been foreseen, yet all the stories about the influenza tended to minimize the scope of this Midwestern outbreak. Perhaps the spirit of positivism found so useful in the war effort was being pressed into service in dealing with the Spanish flu. Did officials see a necessity to maintain a picture of good health in the city even in the face of an epidemic that was afflicting much of the nation? Was the conflict between balancing the necessity for adequate warning with need for good morale already on the minds of some officials?

The war, however, was what most people were thinking about, and so it is not unusual to find individuals in the United States who related the flu to the German enemy. Germ warfare was perceived as a threat in 1918. Lieutenant Colonel Philip S. Doane, head of the Health and Sanitation Section of the Emergency Fleet Corporation, was in Chicago for a speech on

---

[10] *Chicago Tribune*, Sept. 19, 1918.

[11] *Ibid.*

September 18. News reports quoted him under the heading "Started by Hun Agents?"[12]

> It is quite possible that the epidemic was started by Huns sent ashore by boche submarine commanders. We know men have been ashore from such submarines. It would be quite easy for one of these German agents to turn loose Spanish influenza germs in a theater or other places where large numbers of people are assembled. The Germans have started epidemics in Europe, and there is no reason why they should be particularly gentle to America.

Somewhat more vigorous efforts followed. On September 20, the entire Great Lakes base was quarantined, and Chicago's First Deputy Superintendent of Police, Morgan Collins suggested that the city stencil signs reading "Don't Spit" at every intersection. Acting Chief of Police Alcock said the police were still "crusading" against the nuisance of spitting. An anti-tuberculosis campaign had been mounted the previous spring. Now there was another reason to stop spitting. A headline read "Anti-Spitting Campaign to Keep Down Grip."[13] Would the threat of deadly disease make the populace change its patterns of behavior? A *Tribune* editorial warned against kissing during the epidemic because that was an obvious method of "passing it around." Saluting was promoted in place of shaking hands.

By September 21, there were about 400 cases in Chicago proper. Community events were being called off or postponed. Dr. Robertson, confined for a few days to Jefferson Park Hospital (reportedly with a case of neuritis) was quoted in the *Tribune* as saying "... Everything possible is being done to prevent a further spread. I see no cause for public alarm, but every one developing any symptom should be careful."[14] The *Herald and Examiner*

---

[12] *Ibid.* The theory that the Germans were using germ warfare was widespread in America, despite the fact that Germany was suffering from the same pandemic. Crosby believes the flu may have so weakened the German army that its last drive failed for lack of healthy soldiers. Alfred W. Crosby, *Epidemic and Peace, 1918* (Westport, CT, 1976), 7-9.

[13] *Chicago Tribune*, Sept. 24, 1918. The spirit of volunteerism was alive in the American Protective League: it offered services as unofficial policemen in enforcing the anti-spitting ordinance. *Chicago Daily News*, Sept. 30, 1918.

[14] *Chicago Tribune*, Sept. 21, 1918.

for that day reported 2,000 cases at Great Lakes, and printed a warning from Army Surgeon General William Gorgas that the epidemic in military camps was spreading. A *Herald* writer quoted Royal Copeland, New York City health commissioner, as saying that a new organism had been revealed as the cause of this disease.[15]

Secretary of the Navy Josephus Daniels, coming to Chicago to celebrate the Illinois Centennial and Liberty week, believed the facilities at the Great Lakes Station were sufficient to control the epidemic there. Captain Moffett, although ill with flu, tried to calm anxious relatives by saying that the health situation at his camp looked bad only because of the contrast between the present situation and the previous very good health record. The track and field meet at the Station was not cancelled or postponed. The first day was a qualified success. Illinois Athletic club runner Joie Ray won the mile race, but only a fraction of the crowd expected was on hand to cheer him.

The Health Department *Bulletin* of September 21 certainly did not emphasize the threat of epidemic. It merely stated that influenza was "somewhat prevalent in various places in this country. A few cases are now reported in Chicago. This disease is dangerous because pneumonia and other diseases often follow an attack and result fatally."[16] Press releases from the military continued to be sanguine. Even though headlines on the 23rd read "100 Sailors at Great Lakes Die of Influenza" and "4,500 Cases Now Under Treatment, 1,000 Serious," Navy Surgeon Mink was quoted as saying "We have the Spanish influenza situation well in hand now." People were imagining they had the flu when they really had a cold, the report went on. Still, John Philip Sousa's Battalion Band, caught at the base when the quarantine was announced, was not allowed to leave on its Liberty Loan tour. The *Tribune* praised the young men who had died of flu at Great Lakes, saying they had "given their lives to their nation," but another article seemed to shrug off the whole situation with a laugh: "Lassies Lonely as Grip

---

[15]*Chicago Herald and Examiner*, Sept. 21, 1918.

[16]Chicago Health Department *Bulletin*, 12 (Sept. 21, 1918): 167.

Keeps Jackies Away." One writer called it a "so-called influenza epidemic...."[17]

The city Health Department was by this time beginning to take some steps, however. Dr. Robertson declared influenza a reportable disease, effective September 23. All city doctors were to notify the City Health Department of confirmed cases of flu. (Table 7.3 indicates the reporting from several weeks prior to Robertson's declaration until May 3, 1919.) On the 24th the Department began in earnest to prosecute its campaign for adequate heat in rental apartments. Renters were urged to bring complaints to the Commissioner's attention. Recalcitrant landlords were said to be excusing their "frugality" in the face of the inordinately cold weather, citing wartime austerity measures.

Table 7.3

Weekly Morbidity and Mortality Reports
(Aug. 3, 1918 to May 3, 1919)

	Influenza		*Pneumonia*	
Week Ending	*Cases*	*Deaths*	*Cases*	*Deaths*
Aug 3	0	0	18	21
Aug 10	0	2	13	19
Aug 17	0	0	23	19
Aug 24	0	1	33	19
Aug 31	0	2	9	13
Sept 7	0	0	26	17
Sept 14	0	1	27	15
Sept 21	7	0	34	24
Sept 28	193	17	153	74
Oct 5	2,210	171	988	246
Oct 12	7,743	571	2,327	476
Oct 19	10,791	1,242	3,276	863
Oct 26	9,747	1,541	2,968	826
Nov 2	4,943	1,014	1,975	456
Nov 9	1,559	488	926	250
Nov 16	714	235	602	155
Nov 23	728	146	462	105
Nov 30	641	148	264	69
Dec 7	1,716	159	487	103
Dec 14	2,869	269	672	158
Dec 21	2,722	337	916	159

[17] *Chicago Tribune*, Sept. 24, 1918.

Table 7.3
(Continued)

Weekly Morbidity and Mortality Reports
(Aug. 3, 1918 to May 3, 1919)

	Influenza		*Pneumonia*	
Week Ending	*Cases*	*Deaths*	*Cases*	*Deaths*
Dec 28	1,360	281	567	158
Jan 4	868	179	547	142
Jan 11	926	166	473	103
Jan 18	1,042	190	515	138
Jan 25	1,330	183	551	157
Feb 1	866	152	461	125
Feb 8	543	102	363	92
Feb 15	554	100	402	135
Feb 22	498	102	482	131
Mar 1	480	92	451	138
Mar 8	349	88	434	125
Mar 15	419	99	389	133
Mar 22	324	90	390	131
Mar 29	193	80	324	119
Apr 5	155	58	297	112
Apr 12	144	40	273	95
Apr 19	90	21	279	102
Apr 26	53	18	223	63
May 3	67	25	172	63

Source: Chicago Health Department *Bulletin*, Aug. 3, 1918-May 3, 1919.

An optimistic outlook was still being promoted in regard to the epidemic, however. A front-page *Tribune* cartoon featured a picture of the Allies advancing in Europe. The caption read, "Speaking of Epidemics. . . The Influenza Attacks are Nothing compared to the Allied Attacks." The Health Commissioner said he could see no reason to fear that Chicago would be swept by a severe epidemic. He said the public had been told how to protect itself and he foresaw no danger.[18] In the *Daily News* of September 24 he had been quoted as saying, "There is no epidemic in Chicago. If there wasn't trouble from influenza at Great Lakes and the army camps, nothing would be thought of the few cases in Chicago. The danger is no greater than

[18]*Ibid.*, Sept. 25, 1918.

ordinary at this time of year." This was a remarkable statement in the light of reports coming from East Coast cities and the army cantonments at the time, where hundreds were dying each day.

Dr. C. St. Clair Drake of the Illinois Department of Health issued an order on September 26 forbidding public funerals and asking Illinois doctors, nurses, and druggists to report all cases of flu to his office. But while draft officials were postponing a call for 142,000 men and Massachusetts was urgently requesting medical aid from other states, Dr. Robertson insisted that the Spanish flu in the Chicago area, while worse in the suburbs, was not alarming. He recommended that city-dwellers wear gauze masks. "Many cases are merely colds," said one article.[19]

September 28 was, however, something of a turning point in official action against flu. Prompted by a telegram from Washington, Dr. A. J. Ochsner, of the Illinois Council for National Defense, appointed the Illinois Influenza Commission. While it was strictly advisory, this eight-member commission was to coordinate flu preparedness and relief work. With the appointment of this committee, public health activities seemed to shift into a higher gear. The flu had been in the Chicago area for three weeks by this time. More and more people had the illness, or knew someone who had it. The *Tribune* of Sunday, September 29, carried five front-page articles about the epidemic, and the next day the *Herald and Examiner* joined the outcry quoting the new commission as follows:[20]

> We are confronted by an epidemic of influenza which will affect more than half our population in all probability. There is a shortage of physicians, nurses and hospital accommodations. . . .The health and efficiency of the civilian population must be maintained. It is the patriotic duty of every citizen to avoid influenza. Keep in good health.

The Commission requested city nurses to ride the elevated and surface lines with gauze masks over mouth and nose in an effort to educate

---

[19]*Ibid.*, Sept. 28, 1918.

[20]*Chicago Herald and Examiner*, Sept. 30, 1918.

the public on the use of masks.[21] Dr. Robertson was delegated to travel to Washington, D.C. to get the latest news from the East Coast and the United States Public Health Service on how to deal with the epidemic and to ask about a vaccine.

The Chicago Medical Society, speaking to its members through its weekly *Bulletin* of September 28, sounded a somber note:

> "Word comes that some Eastern States are crying for aid to combat a disease, which is swift in its stroke, has a high mortality, and of which we know but little. . . . Preparation is the greater part of the battle. . . . It is well for the profession to lay its fences for the onslaught. We have every reason to expect an attack. Forewarned is forearmed. . . ."[22]

The city seems to have awakened to the peril. Former Health Commissioner Dr. W. A. Evans, a member of the Influenza Commission, began writing articles about prevention and treatment in his "How to Keep Well" newspaper column. Stories at this time varied widely in their treatment of the epidemic ranging from suggesting that there was no cause for alarm to reporting that the Commission was searching for vacant buildings in which to open hospital annexes.

On September 30, the City Health Department issued an order to street-car and elevated train companies to clean, disinfect, and generally renovate their cars. The Department also began publishing hand-outs about the flu for distribution at the city's 324 schools. Two days earlier, the Department had called a meeting with city social welfare agencies to consider whether to keep the schools open. Some eastern cities had closed theirs, as had some North Shore communities. The consensus was to keep Chicago schools open, thus keeping children from congregating in the cold. The school inspection service of physicians and nurses which was employed by the Health Department could survey each class at assigned schools to discover incipient cases of flu, and could more easily educate the students as

---

[21]*Ibid.*

[22]In that issue of the C.M.S. *Bulletin*, the Society offered a free examination of all sputa in suspected cases of Spanish flu, looking for what was mistakenly believed the cause of the illness, Pfeiffer's bacillus.

to proper prevention and treatment. As the epidemic progressed, schools were ordered to leave all windows open through the entire day for better ventilation. To avoid chilling faculty and students, buildings were to be super-heated. Dry sweeping floors was forbidden in an effort to reduce the spread of dust.

A quarantine of flu cases was promulgated beginning on September 30, and Cook County Hospital was quarantined. It had admitted more than 60 cases on the preceding Saturday alone. This institution, the municipal hospital for city patients unable to pay for private care, admitted more than 2,000 flu patients between the 23rd of September and the 29th of October. Of these, 642 died, a mortality of about 31%. The age range of highest mortality was 25 to 30 years. Hospitalized pregnant women suffered an even higher mortality due to flu and pneumonia; almost half (46%) died. More than 50 nurses at Cook County Hospital became ill as did 12 resident physicians. Three nurses died. The epidemic "seriously crippled the medical and more especially the nursing staff of the hospital."[23]

Some feared the city's hospitals would be overwhelmed by the crisis. They were, after all, already burdened with war-wounded and many physicians and nurses had gone into the Armed Services. One doctor called his hospital a "war-crippled institution." The staffs at other hospitals fared no better than Cook County's. Three nurses died at West Side Hospital, and forty were ill at Presbyterian. Dr. Drake directed that all hospital attendants in flu cases wear medicated masks. Various communities commandeered large homes and other institutions for use as temporary hospitals.

On the first day of October, newspapers gave advice to "Seek good air, shun bad air," and to stay away from crowds and places of public assembly.[24] The *Daily News* carried an estimate of 12,000 to 15,000 flu deaths in Chicago. Dr. Drake was quoted as saying he had no wish to spread a panic, but in his opinion it was best that the public know what danger it was facing. Illinois Governor Frank O. Lowden ordered all public buildings in the state,

[23]John W. Nuzum, *et al.*, "1918 Pandemic Influenza and Pneumonia in a Large Civil Hospital," reprinted in *The Illinois Medical Journal*, 105 (Dec., 1976): 612-16.

[24]*Chicago Tribune*, Oct. 1, 1918.

including the Joliet State Penitentiary, closed to visitors. City street-cleaning workers were issued masks.

By early October, the Spanish flu began to leave the Great Lakes Naval Training Station. Captain Moffett was able to say that after two weeks of increase, the number of cases in his camp was decreasing. But now morbidity and mortality statistics for Chicago began to reflect the severity of the epidemic: in three days, September 28-30, 44 deaths in the city were attributed to flu and pneumonia. October 1, 370 new cases were reported, with 59 deaths. Further expressions of concern appeared. A Health Department doctor was quoted as saying that hospital bed space was already filled.[25] This disease appeared to require nursing especially, since there were no drug therapies or other medical interventions a doctor alone could administer. One physician wrote, "The value of good nursing cannot be overestimated," while another said nurses were more valuable than doctors in this epidemic.[26]

The American Red Cross urged graduate nurses to apply to local Red Cross bureaus for immediate duty. "We are swamped with calls for nurses to go to army camps and cantonments, civilian hospitals, and to the homes where the victims of the epidemic are lying ill."[27] Later, the A.R.C. issued pleas for any women with time and inclination to help.

> "Nursing service will win the local war against Spanish influenza. The need for nurses is great--beyond anything the community has ever known. . . . We appeal. . . to *all* women, regardless of their lack of professional training, who are willing to give time and service in the stricken homes. . . .who can give a few hours of time each day in the ordinary household duties such as putting homes in order and preparing foods."[28]

---

[25]*Ibid.*, Oct. 2, 1918.

[26]W.W.G. Maclachlan, "The Treatment of Influenza," in The University of Pittsburgh School of Medicine, *Studies on Epidemic Influenza* (Pittsburgh, 1919), 83; Crosby, 6-7.

[27]American Red Cross, Chicago Chapter *Bulletin*, 11 (Oct. 4, 1918): 4.

[28]*Ibid.*, 3.

The Influenza Commission requested the city Health Department to take daily counts of beds available in the city hospitals, and continued to consider opening temporary hospitals in vacant buildings. The Department issued an order excluding all visitors from hospitals except in emergencies, and ordered theater owners to bar patrons with colds, sneezes, or coughs. Posters were placed at theater entrances:

> INFLUENZA FREQUENTLY COMPLICATED WITH PNEUMONIA IS PREVALENT AT THIS TIME THROUGHOUT AMERICA THIS THEATER IS CO-OPERATING WITH THE DEPARTMENT OF HEALTH YOU MUST DO THE SAME
>
> IF YOU HAVE A COLD AND ARE COUGHING AND SNEEZING, DO NOT ENTER THIS THEATRE GO HOME AND GO TO BED UNTIL YOU ARE WELL
>
> Coughing, Sneezing or Spitting Will Not Be Permitted in the Theatre. In Case You must cough or Sneeze, do so in your own hand-kerchief, and if the Coughing or Sneezing Persists Leave the Theatre at Once.
>
> This Theatre has agreed to co-operate with the Department of Health in Disseminating the truth about Influenza, and thus serve a Great educational purpose.

HELP US KEEP CHICAGO THE HEALTHIEST CITY IN THE WORLD
JOHN DILL ROBERTSON
COMMISSIONER OF HEALTH

On October 2, a four-column headline on page 17 of the *Tribune* announced: "88,000 flu cases in camps of U.S." The article featured photographs of a street sweeper, an intern, and a County Hospital nurse wearing masks. On the same page, a former city health commissioner Dr. Charles Whalen predicted 15,000 flu deaths in the city, with 60% to 70% of the population ill. The following day's column by Dr. Evans described the symptoms and common treatments, but concluded, "It appears to be so easily communicable that no preventive measures offer much."[29] Still, Commissioner Robertson held to the view that there would not be a large death toll. He said estimates frightened the public. He urged precautions, but thought that the disease would run its course in Chicago within six weeks, with little or no increase in deaths. October 4th's *Tribune* editorialized against panic, urging precaution instead of fear. "We are not heading into a cataclysm and the last thing we can profitably use is a feeling of panic."

In an exercise in public prophylaxis, Dr. Robertson requested Acting Police Chief Alcock to order the arrest of all persistent coughers and sneezers who failed to cover their faces with handkerchiefs. The newspaper carried this announcement: "If the person approached by the policeman promises to obey the instructions in the future he will be allowed to go; but if he talks back to the policeman he will be taken into custody." Later, said the paper, he will be dismissed with a warning lecture by a magistrate. The story added the comment that actual arrests were unlikely, since their legality was uncertain.[30] On October 6, however, street cars, elevated stations, and public buildings as well as theaters were told to display warning cards bearing in large letters: "SPITTING ARRESTED AND PROSECUTED." Thirty-three persons were arrested, tried, and convicted of spitting on elevated platforms, but the penalty was minimal. Municipal Court Judge John Haas fined them each $1.00.[31]

Pastors of all Chicago churches were asked to request parishioners with coughs or sneezes to stay at home. However, the Commission expressed the desire that nothing be done to interfere with the morale of the community. Churches were not ordered closed, although they were asked to leave windows open for better ventilation and to limit the length of their services. The Church Federation Council offered to close all its member churches. A few congregations did so on their own initiative. At Kenwood

---

[29] *Chicago Tribune*, Oct. 3, 1918.

[30] *Ibid.*, Oct. 4, 1918; *Chicago Daily News*, Oct. 3, 1918.

[31] *Chicago Tribune*, Oct. 6, 1918. The *Herald and Examiner* for Oct. 23 reported that twenty-five spitters were each fined $1.00 and costs the day before.

Church on Greenwood Avenue the sermon for Sunday, October 20, was titled "Staying the Plague," and at Wicker Park Lutheran the pastor spoke of "The Present Judgement."[32] Archbishop Mundelein issued regulations on October 17 to the Roman Catholic archdiocese suspending evening services and forbidding long sermons. Church attendance reported declined to one-third or one-half of normal.[33]

October 6 was Liberty Loan Sunday, the opening day for Liberty Week, and Dr. Robertson on Monday expressed the idea that according to daily reports the epidemic was waning in the city as the weather warmed. The *Tribune* agreed that the city was holding its own. However, despite the warmer weather and expressions of hope, the epidemic was not in decline. Morbidity and mortality reports confirmed that it was spreading. What further steps would city officials take? On October 11, the Influenza Commission had a long debate about a general closing order. Opinion was divided. Commissioner Robertson was against general closing. In the *Report* he compiled after the epidemic, he wrote:

> In a great city like Chicago, in which one fortieth [sic] of the population of the entire nation resides, and in war time, when it is absolutely essential. . . to keep the arteries of business open, the plan of closing business and stopping commerce could not be considered for one moment.[34]

What emerged from this first debate was a very limited closing order: funeral attendance (already affected by an earlier state order) was limited, and dance halls were closed. The Commission reportedly saw the close contact of dancing as dangerous. Dancers would be working up a sweat which would be followed by chilling. Smoking on street cars was also prohibited. The doors to front "vestibules" of the city's 3,000 surface cars, where smoking had previously been allowed, were to be propped open for better air circulation, and now these vestibules could be used to

---

[32]*Chicago Tribune*, Oct. 20, 1918.

[33]*Ibid.*, Oct. 13, 16, 17, 19, 21, 1918; Robertson, 74-75.

[34]*Ibid.*, 45.

accommodate more passengers, avoiding overcrowding and allowing for more "fresh air." Smokers, in addition, had the habit of spitting on the floors of the cars, and the no-smoking order went to the issue of spitting as well. "No Smoking" was to be the rule on the city's 1,700 elevated cars also. The usual smoking cars would be devoted to general passenger traffic, thus better distributing the ridership. New train schedules were to be worked out to ease peak loads and prevent overcrowding. It was also hoped that a way could be found to arrange staggered quitting times for downtown businesses. Shoppers were urged to leave for home before the workers, in any case.

Saturday, October 12, was Liberty Day! Between 100,000 and 200,000 people were expected for a march. Secretary of the Navy Josephus Daniels and Ex-President Theodore Roosevelt were to be on hand to raise public enthusiasm for war bond sales. The parade was not ordered postponed or cancelled. Marchers were advised, however, to go home, remove all clothing, rub the body dry and put on warm clothing afterward, and to try not to get chilled on the way home. Elevated and surface lines were asked to heat cars in the afternoon. One writer concluded his advice with "Take a laxative when you reach home and you will minimize your chances of catching the disease."[35]

During the week following the march, the Commission met at least three times. More-inclusive closing orders now appeared necessary, as the death rate from influenza and pneumonia had jumped from 8.37 per 1,000 for the week ending October 5 to 21.01 per 1,000 for the week ending on the 12th. On the 14th the Commission formulated a general closing order. The police were to see to the closing of all theaters, skating rinks, moving picture shows, night schools, and lodge halls. The order was executed efficiently; the *Tribune* on Wednesday reported that the Loop was "deserted last night." The only outside activity after 9:00 p.m. was the fire department hosing down the streets. Restaurants were almost empty. The city was "lightless, theaterless, and danceless," according to one reporter.[36]

---

[35] *Chicago Tribune*, Oct. 13, 1918.

[36] *Ibid.*, Oct. 16, 1918. This order presented an opportunity to the Illinois Women's Christian Temperance Union. Its President, Helen L. Hood, sent letters to Mayor Thompson and

The closing order was interpreted by some in the Health Department as more than merely prevention. It would act as a preservative as well. The Department *Bulletin* for October 19, seeming at last to recognize the severity of the threat, yet still using positive terms (in war-time imagery), stated that the closing order was a good thing because it meant that "people will be preserving their vital powers." By not going out to a theater in the evenings, reasoned the writer, people will probably go to bed earlier, and will thus "conserve their physical powers and energies for the next day's battle of life."[37] People were urged not only to stay home in the evenings but also to refrain from using the telephone. The telephone company in Chicago bought advertisements requesting people to limit calls since so many operators were out sick.[38]

On October 18, the closure was extended to such gatherings as banquets, conventions, lectures, debates, lodges, labor union meetings, and athletic contests. Music, cabarets (floor shows), and other entertainments were stopped, as were all billiard, pool, and bowling matches.

Quackery and patent medicine were quick to take profit. In South Chicago two "doctors" used a snake charmer to draw a crowd so they could sell their flu decoction, until police dispersed the assembly. Patent medicine manufacturers capitalized on the circumstances, advertising in the dailies. "Father John's Medicine" was claimed to be able to build "strength to resist grip germs" and was a "Safe preventive. Free from alcohol." "Kondon's Catarrhal Jelly" ads bore a "personal offer to those who fear Spanish influenza." Buyers could get their money back if not satisfied (and if still alive). This advertisement claimed that many doctors were recommending such a jelly as Kondon's for a "soothing antiseptic for inside the nose and head."[39]

Commissioner Robertson urging that saloons be included in the closing order. The city's saloons remained open.

[37]Chicago Health Department *Bulletin*, 12 (Oct. 19, 1918): 183.

[38]*Chicago Tribune*, Oct. 17, 1918.

[39]*Chicago Daily News*, Oct. 10, 1918; *Chicago Tribune*, Oct. 17, 1918.

Other business interests sought to capitalize on people's fear of flu. The Truax company of 141 North Wabash Avenue offered gauze masks to industrial companies at an individual rate of 10 cents each, or in bulk at $12.00 per gross. Lysol sought to use its ads to sell its disinfectant and at the same time educate the citizenry toward better hygiene: "Epidemics are born of dirt and ignorance," the ad said. "Disinfect your home regularly and thoroughly with Lysol."[40] According to another advertiser, a person's diet could affect how well he recovered from a case of flu. "A recuperative diet in influenza. Horlick's Malted Milk; very digestible."[41]

The people were not without traditional remedies. Mrs. Anna Olds Woodson of South Chicago had a fumigative remedy which she kindly sent to the War Department. Her advice was to finely chop red peppers and boil them with all doors and windows closed, letting the influenza patient inhale the fumes. Repeat if needed. A letter to the Editor of the *Tribune* announced that an excellent preventive was to eat a small raw onion in the forenoon, at noon, and at night. This would prevent contracting influenza, or any other disease. "Garlic is even better," the writer concluded. Some stories had it that removal of tonsils or extraction of teeth, or even inhalation of chloroform, would cure the flu.[42] Too much of the latter would certainly terminate the case.

News of a possibly effective vaccine to prevent contracting influenza spurred the Influenza Commission to appoint a citizen's committee to seek ways to raise funds for production. The committee included such notables as J. Ogden Armour, William Wrigley, and Louis Kuppenheimer. Dr. E. C. Rosenow of the Mayo Foundation was interviewed on October 16 about the vaccine he had devised, and the decision was made to have the Chicago Health Department laboratories manufacture and distribute his vaccine.

---

[40]*Ibid.*, Oct. 18, 1918.

[41]*Ibid.*, Oct. 19, 1918.

[42]Joseph. E. Persico, "The Great Swine Flu Epidemic of 1918," *American Heritage*, (June, 1976): 83.

The City Council voted $18,000 for the production of the vaccine, but it did not become available for general use until after October 21.[43]

The papers on October 19 told of a survey of city hospitals revealing a considerable number of empty beds, seeming to confirm the suspicion that some private hospitals were refusing indigent patients. Many hospitals, wrote Robertson in his *Report*, "Showed a commendable spirit of cooperation" by setting aside a number of beds for indigent flu cases, allowing ambulances to take such cases to the nearest hospital, "obviating a long haul to Cook County Hospital." On October 5, the Commissioner had written to all Chicago hospitals in this regard:

> "I want to bespeak your continued cooperation with the Department of Health. It is my judgement that you should not refuse to admit influenza and pneumonia patients, to the limit of the capacity of your nursing service. If we all pull together in this matter, this epidemic will be quickly stamped out, and the hospitals then can resume their regular procedures."[44]

Had the city's hospitals reached maximum capacity early in the epidemic? There was an impression that they had, but the Progressive search for equal treatment for both rich and poor seems to have been left with a nagging doubt. A first survey of 63 of the city's 90-some hospitals showed 7,190 patients, 803 of whom were flu cases, and 1,675 beds were empty. The second survey, reported on October 19, seemed to indicate that the hospitals were "not utilizing their available space for influenza. . . ." Robertson called a meeting of hospital representatives for October 20.[45]

The meeting was inconclusive. While admitting they had space, private hospitals argued that they lacked nursing staff to care for more

[43]Robertson, 81-83. The efficacy of the influenza vaccines was by no means uncontested at the time. Formulas like Dr. Rosenow's from the Mayo Foundation in Minnesota were considered by many to be of uncertain value. One commentator expressed the opinion that the "greatest value of vaccine therapy was in the fact that it reduced fluphobia, as it has been clearly demonstrated that worry and fear had to be controlled during the epidemic." Quoted in George M. Price, "Influenza--Destroyer and Teacher: A General Confession by the Public Health Authorities of a Continent," *The Survey*, 41 (Dec. 21, 1918): 367-69.

[44]Robertson, 68-69.

[45]*Chicago Tribune*, Oct. 20, 1918; Robertson, 68, 70.

patients. Suspicion remained, however, that the private hospitals were not sharing the burden of care for non-paying influenza patients. Robertson stated on the 23rd that those shown to be refusing treatment would face "drastic measures," perhaps even loss of license.[46]

Morbidity and mortality in the city peaked in mid-October and began slowly to decline, although weekly totals (see Table 7.3) would not show a significant drop until the second week in November. The Department *Bulletin* for October 26 announced that the epidemic was passing. Officials promptly turned to rescinding the closing orders. This they did in stages. On October 29, music and entertainments in restaurants were allowed, and reopening of the city's 403 theaters was made contingent upon general clean-up and renovation. On November 4, dance halls and lodge halls were allowed to reopen after an inspection. Social functions, athletic contests, and other previously banned public gatherings were again permitted, but the anti-smoking order was not lifted. "So long as there is smoking on cars it will be impossible to prevent expectoration," wrote Robertson. Where there was sputum on floors, disease would be carried.[47]

Chicago emerged from the epidemic of Spanish flu with a better health record than many other large cities in the United States. From September 21 to November 16, 1918, there were approximately 37,900 recorded cases of influenza in the city, and 13,000 cases of pneumonia. The total reported morbidity from Spanish flu was about 51,000, and total mortality was about 8,500. Yet these figures must be considered in relation to the relatively short time the epidemic afflicted the city. The death rate for Chicago during the epidemic went as high as 63 per 1,000. By way of comparison, Philadelphia's rate reached 156, Baltimore's 147, and Pittsburgh's 99. St. Louis fared comparatively well, with a death rate of only 28 per 1,000.[48]

---

[46]*Chicago Tribune*, Oct. 23, 1918.

[47]Robertson, 97-99.

[48]*Ibid.*, 5, 28.

Was the Spanish flu selective in terms of race or ethnicity? In his *Report* after the epidemic, Robertson stated that the relative increases in deaths of "colored" and white populations were quite different, with whites showing a 2,610% increase over an average of October, 1917, and September, 1918, while coloreds showed an increase of only 1,400%. In addition, Robertson reported an analysis of ethnic backgrounds of influenza and pneumonia fatalities. The report concluded that in Chicago the greatest relative increase in deaths was among the Bohemian, Lithuanian, and Polish nationalities, and the lowest relative increases were among the native born. How much these results had to do with housing and population density remains a question.[49] Dr. Edwin O. Jordan, in his *Epidemic Influenza: A Survey* (1927) corroborated Robertson's conclusion about relatively lower total morbidity among black Americans. He qualified this by stating that blacks in the U.S. had had a higher case fatality, but a lower attack rate. Jordan indicated that Italian-Americans had suffered more than other nationalities, and stated that (true to a centuries-old pattern) American Indians had had an unusually high mortality.[50]

While it is impossible conclusively to determine what effects, if any, the actions taken against flu had on its progress or severity, it is likely that sensible preventive measures had some positive results. Certainly the city's Health Department, once it had decided that there was indeed a threat, exerted intensive efforts. In addition to the activities already described, the Department asked factories to have a sick call each morning, and department employees surveyed schools, homes, and businesses in the city's seventeen health districts.[51] The survey work among the homes of a neighborhood, undertaken by volunteer workers, seems to have been important, perhaps more so in some areas of the city than in others. The Visiting Nurse Association report indicated some resistance to or fear of medical professionals, especially among the immigrant population, and in the poorer

---

[49] *Ibid.*, 26--Tables 9 and 10, 35-37.

[50] Edwin O. Jordan, *Epidemic Influenza: A Survey* (Chicago, 1927), 244-47.

[51] Robertson, 59-61.

neighborhoods. Mary E. Westphal, the Visiting Nurse Superintendent in Chicago wrote this anecdote about the Spanish flu in one neighborhood:[52]

> The ghetto was a hotbed of influenza and pneumonia. People watched at the window, at the doors, then beckoned us to come in, although our gowns and masks frightened some. On one of the coldest, rainiest days which we had, the nurse met on the sidewalk in front of a home, an 8-year-old boy, barefoot and in his nightdress. She quickly saw that he was delirious and coaxing him back into the house, she found his father sitting beside the stove, his head in his hands, two children in one bed, the mother and a two weeks old baby in another. She questioned the man, who was nearly crazed because, as he told her, he had just given his wife, a pneumonia patient, a spoonful of camphorated oil instead of castor oil. He had been up all night and day caring for the wife and children, all with temperatures above 104°. The nurse sent for the doctor, administered to the woman, bathed all the patients and sent the youngest child to the hospital, where he died a few days later. Four of our families lost both mothers and fathers. We tried hard to save a 28-year-old mother of four children with a baby 9 months old. She was pregnant and died on the 11th day.

Also aiding the Health Department in medical relief work were the charitable institutions of the city. The United Charities, with approximately 85 field workers made about 2,500 calls on families having flu. In addition to its official role as nursing coordinator for the nation during the epidemic, the American Red Cross spent over $500,000 for influenza care nation-wide, and in the Chicago area served more than 1,000 families with food and medical aid, opening 11 emergency kitchens around the city.[53] They worked with a staff of 50 graduate nurses and nearly 300 volunteers. The A.R.C. distributed about 43,000 gauze masks through their field workers. Other groups helped as well. The Infant Welfare Society cared for more than 4,000 families in the city, and the Jewish Aid Society, which had 14 field workers and one trained

---

[52]Quoted in Hoehling, 148.

[53]*Chicago Tribune*, Oct. 19, 1918.

nurse, worked at the West Side Dispensary to provide bedside care and meals at the Society's expense.[54]

The Visiting Nurse Association reported an increase in activity of 400% because of the flu. Their report on the Spanish flu included notice that the epidemic revealed a shortage of everything, including "intelligent relatives," and especially nurses. It also cast light on the need, as it was then seen, for improved family and personal hygiene. The V.N.A. report indicated a desire to explore the possibility of a system of health insurance.[55]

Hull House, Jane Addams' settlement house in Halsted Street, served as a kitchen for indigent influenza patients and their families, as did the Chicago Commons, the near-north settlement begun by Graham Taylor. Workers from the Commons were used as investigators by the Red Cross to screen phone calls for aid. In the Commons' 1918 Annual Report, Mr. Taylor wrote: "The after effects of the influenza will be felt in family life for some time. Motherless children, heavy debts incurred, impaired general health--these problems will last over many a year."[56]

> Several major responses to this epidemic seem to stand out. Dependence upon community services increased. Now that the urban area had grown to such great proportions, it had become imperative that organization triumph over independence, that the special services seen as necessary to progress and civilization be promoted. "Co-operate with the Department of Health in all that it urges and advises," said the Health Department *Bulletin*. Chicago has never been defeated in anything that it has undertaken to do. It has now taken in hand the task of fighting this threatened epidemic of influenza. The Commissioner of Health believes with the hearty co-operation of the people of Chicago, it will not fail now, . . . Let us be up and doing to win this fight against influenza.[57]

---

[54]Robertson, 64-67.

[55]The Visiting Nurse Association of Chicago, "Twenty-Ninth Annual Report" (Chicago, 1918), 43-46.

[56]Chicago Commons, "Annual Report of the Work of Chicago Commons for the Year Ending Sept. 30, 1919." Manuscript, Collection of the Chicago Historical Society. Not paginated.

[57]Chicago Health Department *Bulletin*, 12 (Oct. 12, 1918): 181.

Another response was the rejection of fear and worry. *The Survey* magazine quoted Commissioner Robertson as saying, "It is our duty to keep the people from fear. Worry kills more people than the epidemic. For my part, let them wear a rabbit's foot on a watch-chain if they want it and if it will help them get rid of the psychological action of fear."[58] The *Literary Digest* quoted the proclamation, ". . . fear is our first enemy. . . . whether he fights a German or a germ, the man who worries is already half beaten. . . . from battle to disease the cool fighter wins."[59] And the Chicago Health Department *Bulletin* boldly advised, ". . . there is no need for panic. There are many cases where fear rather than disease kills. Don't be apprehensive. In other words, don't be afraid."[60] The admonitions against fear and anxiety fit well into the picture of an America believing in itself, confident of its future and striving ever upwards toward bigger and better. There was no room for irrational fear in the new world into which America was heading in 1918.

Not until a long time after the outbreak of the disease on the East Coast, and after the first cases in the area, was official Chicago convinced that serious measures must be taken to combat the Spanish flu. The epidemic had peaked before closing orders were issued. Was Commissioner Robertson afraid of the business interests in the city, and thus hesitant to publicize the threat or agree to a general closing order? Others were ready early in the epidemic to speak in terms of tens of thousands of deaths. Yet when action was taken, it was sensible and appropriate.

One thing that seems to stand out in assessing the city's responses to the flu is the media's role in promoting a "positive attitude" toward the threat--carrying stories that spoke reassuringly, editorializing about "Doing your bit," rejecting fear and worry, increasingly depending on professional care and advice.

---

[58]*The Survey*, 41 (Dec. 21, 1918): 268.

[59]Quoted in *The Literary Digest*, 59 (Oct. 12, 1918): 13-14.

[60]Chicago Department of Health *Bulletin*, 12 (Oct. 12, 1918): 181.

In the end, it appears that officials largely succeeded in balancing the threat of the epidemic with the threat of a panic (or a business slow-down). The worst that can be said is that private hospitals may not have been carrying their share of the influenza and pneumonia cases. No mass exodus or incidents of looting that might have accompanied earlier epidemics characterized Chicago's response to the flu. And neither were there any official public services for contrition and prayer; the only large gathering was for the Liberty Loan parade.

Chapter 8: San Diego

Richard Peterson

The war years, with the congregation and movement of soldiers and refugees from place to place, created ideal conditions for the spread of influenza. American soldiers returning from the European front apparently carried the virus to the east coast. However, Colonel Philip S. Doane, head of the health and sanitation section of the Emergency Fleet Corporation in Washington, D.C., a merchant-ship auxiliary created during the war, went so far as to hypothesize that the disease was "brought to the United States by members of German submarines who. . . were reported to have been ashore at New York and other places."[1] Such an allegation was understandable during the emotionally-charged struggle against Germany, which had witnessed the introduction of modern chemical warfare. Indeed the flu was referred to on one occasion as "this new Hun of materia medica."[2] During September, 1918, the flu began to make its presence felt at army camps and naval bases on the eastern seaboard. By September 24, over 20,000 cases had been reported in at at least 25 army camps throughout the entire country, with Massachusetts and New York most seriously affected. Two days later, the number of cases had climbed to over 29,000 with 530 deaths,

---

[1] *San Diego Union*, Sept. 19, 1918. Also see A. A. Hoehling, *The Great Epidemic* (Boston, 1961), 32; and *New York Times*, Sept. 19, 1918.

[2] *San Diego Union*, Sept. 22, 1918. During the war, Germans were vilified by American propagandists as Hun barbarians. The phrase "materia medica" is Latin for medical material.

many from the pneumonia which often accompanied the virus. In fact, every fourth man in the American army camps would suffer from influenza, every twenty-fourth man would develop pneumonia, and every sixty-seventh man would die. At home and abroad, a total of over 621,000 American soldiers caught the flu in 1918.[3]

The disease was not confined to the military. In September, an estimated 85,000 Massachusetts citizens contracted Spanish influenza. Seven hundred died of the flu and pneumonia complications in the last week of the month. In Boston, 202 people succumbed on October 1. New York City reported 3,077 cases in one day, 300 of whom later died. Philadelphia was particularly hard-hit with 700 deaths in a single day and 4,598 fatalities within one week in October. Other large cities from Washington, D.C. to San Francisco, as well as isolated rural areas, were seriously affected as the epidemic swept the country. In the nation's capital undertakers were stationed at the doors of hospitals to remove the deceased promptly enough to make room for the rapid admission of new flu cases. There seemed to be no escape from or defense against this unseen enemy which struck suddenly without warning. Nationwide and worldwide, about 20% of the population caught Spanish influenza, and the death rate was around 3%.[4] In view of the widespread epidemic, what affect did the influenza scourge have on San Diego and how did the local authorities and general public cope with the unprecedented crisis?

Although there are studies of the flu epidemic in other southwestern cities, it has been only barely acknowledged in San Diego. In fact, two recent illustrated general histories of the city fail to mention it.[5] At the same time,

---

[3]*Ibid.*, Sept. 24, 26, 1918; Irwin Ross, "The Great Plague of 1918," *American History Illustrated*, 3 (July, 1968): 12; and Alfred Crosby, Jr., *Epidemic and Peace, 1918* (Westport, CT., 1976), 47, 205-06.

[4]Joseph E. Persico, "The Great Swine Flu Epidemic of 1918," *American Heritage*, 27 (June, 1976): 30-31, 84; *New York Times*, Sept. 29, 1918; *San Diego Union*, Sept. 26, 1918; Hoehling, 51; Crosby, 53, 56-116, 205-07; and Bradford Luckingham, *Epidemic in the Southwest, 1918-1919* (El Paso, 1984), 4.

[5]*Ibid.*, contains information on the epidemic in El Paso, Texas; Albuquerque, New Mexico; and Phoenix and Tucson, Arizona. Also see Richard Melzer, "A Dark and Terrible Moment:

the vast majority of general histories of the United States and regional and state survey histories similarly omit any reference to the national epidemic. Studies of Spanish influenza in the United States emphasize eastern cities like Boston, New York, and Philadelphia and larger cities over 100,000 in population. Therefore, an examination of the flu outbreak in San Diego, a western city with a population of about 70,000 in 1918, would give some balance to this historiographical pattern. The selection of San Diego is appropriate for another reason. It was the site of Camp Kearny, a military facility created in 1917 to train soldiers for overseas duty in World War I. At similar army camps in the east like Camp Devens near Boston and Camp Dix outside of Philadelphia, the flu made early, devastating inroads in the country.[6]

The Spanish Flu Epidemic of 1918 in New Mexico," *New Mexico Historical Review*, 57 (July, 1982): 213-36. The local history books in question are Iris H.W. Engstrand, *San Diego: California's Cornerstone* (Tulsa, Okla., 1980), and Ray Brandes, *San Diego: An Illustrated History* (Los Angeles, 1981). Also see Pierce C. Mullen and Michael L. Nelson, "Montanans and 'the Most Peculiar Disease': The Influenza Epidemic and Public Health, 1918-1919," *Montana: The Magazine of Western History*, 37 (Spring, 1987): 50-61.

[6]The best account of the epidemic on the national and international level, Crosby, *Epidemic and Peace*, documents the spread of influenza in numerous American cities. Crosby includes separate chapters on San Francisco and Philadelphia and draws much of his information from cities with populations in excess of 100,000, arguing that "the best weekly mortality statistics we have are for 45 of the nation's largest cities." See Crosby, 56, 60-61. Hoehling especially emphasizes the epidemic in large Eastern and Midwestern cities, while Richard Collier, *The Plague of the Spanish Lady: The Influenza Pandemic of 1918-1919* (New York, 1974) focuses on the international scene and numerous personal case histories of flu victims. In addition, see William R. Noyes, "Influenza Epidemic, 1918-1919: A Misplaced Chapter in U.S. Social and Institutional History" (Ph.D. diss., University of California, Los Angeles, 1968). This study occasionally refers to the epidemic in Los Angeles, but like the others it concentrates on the reactions to the disease in large Eastern cities. Also useful is Dorothy Ann Pettit, "A Cruel Wind: America Experiences the Pandemic Influenza, 1918-20" (Ph.D. diss., University of New Hampshire, 1976). The latter emphasizes the epidemic abroad and in the eastern United States and offers the provocative thesis that the widespread post-World War I apathy in America was as much the result of the lingering physical effects of influenza as it was a general spiritual depression. In 1920, San Diego's city population officially numbered 74,683. See the *Fourteenth Census of the United States, Population*, 4 vols. (Washington, D.C., 1922), III: 118--Table 10. The estimate of 70,000 for 1918 is suggested by Richard F. Pourade, *The History of San Diego: Gold in the Sun*, 7 vols. (San Diego, 1965), 5 231. For information on the creation of Camp Kearny, see Pourade, 5: 225-227. The epidemic at Camp Devens and Camp Dix is covered in Crosby, 4-11, 25, 28, 40, 67, 71, 91, 171, and 277; and in the *New York Times*, Sept. 15, 21, 23-24, 1918.

Reports of possible Spanish influenza in San Diego came initially from Balboa Park. On September 26, the naval training camp there was quarantined after a number of suspected cases were placed in isolation wards. The next day the Associated Press reported that Camp Kearny was one of many army camps where influenza had appeared, leaving only thirteen camps in the nation free from infection. Medical authorities at Camp Kearny apparently sought to allay fears of public contamination by declaring the flu cases of only the "common garden variety." However, by early October, Camp Kearny, the Balboa naval facility, Fort Rosecrans on Point Loma, and the naval air station on North Island all had been placed under quarantine.[7]

The first official civilian reaction to influenza in San Diego came on October 13. At that time, ten cases of flu were being treated at the county hospital and another seven had been reported among the county jail population. To halt the spread of disease, the city board of health closed all public amusements and facilities indefinitely. The police were authorized to enforce the order against theaters, motion picture houses, churches, dance halls, swimming pools, gymnasiums, schools, bath houses, auction sales, billiard and pool halls, libraries, women's weekly club meetings, and outdoor meetings except Liberty Loan bond gatherings. As a precautionary measure, fire department employees were to spray the nose and throat of those requesting it with a quinine bisulphate solution at various stations throughout the city. The city health board also urged people to spend as much time as possible in the outdoors, since plenty of fresh air and outdoor recreation was recommended as protection against infection.[8]

The first day of the city quarantine passed without serious incident as many citizens sought the alleged health-giving properties of the beaches and back country. In fact, a prominent San Diego physician argued that Spanish influenza germs could not survive in altitudes over 3500 feet. Local residents thus were advised to avoid contagion by taking advantage of the fresh air and

[7]*San Diego Union*, Sept. 26-27, 29; Oct. 4, 12-13, 1918; and *New York Times*, Sept. 27, 1918.

[8]*San Diego Union*, Oct. 13-14, 1918. Although best known as a treatment for malaria, quinine was used for a variety of ailments around the turn of the century.

uncrowded conditions of the nearby Cuyamaca and Laguna Mountains east of the city.[9]

Despite such recommendations and the city quarantine of public facilities, the incidence of influenza rose steadily in October. As of October 14, flu cases numbered 63 with one death. By October 20, total cases in San Diego and the immediate vicinity had increased to 329 with eleven deaths and 77 new cases in a single day. By October 24, as many as 488 cases with 18 deaths had been reported in the city.[10]

In view of the growing health hazard, city medical authorities took further precautionary steps. In cooperation with the local branch of the Red Cross, the spraying of quinine bisulphate was made available at parks, hotels, stores, and other public accommodations. It is doubtful, however, that this preventive had much affect other than to irritate the mucous membranes of the nasal passages, as one cynic complained.[11] On October 18, the board of health urged citizens to wear protective gauze masks--a common practice in the eastern communities of the United States. Those working in close contact with the public such as waiters, barbers, and retail clerks were especially requested to adopt the practice, and the Red Cross sent out appeals for local women to help sew the facial garments at the downtown Red Cross production center. Specific instructions were also issued for those wishing to fashion their own masks at home.[12]

Although there is evidence that many employees in close proximity with the public cooperated with authorities and wore the masks, the general

---

[9] *Ibid.*, Oct. 14, 18, 1918.

[10] *Ibid.*, Oct. 15, 20, 24, 1918.

[11] *Ibid.*, Oct. 16, 1918. See a complaining letter to the editor from W. D. Page of Point Loma, California, *Ibid.*, Nov. 24, 1918. For evidence that the American Public Health Association similarly discounted the value of sprays and gargles as protection against infection, see Wilfred H. Kellogg, *Influenza: A Study of Measures Adopted for the Control of the Epidemic*, California State Board of Health, Special Bulletin No. 31 (Sacramento, 1919), 22-23.

[12] *San Diego Union*, Oct. 18-19, 1918. The California State Board of Health later concluded that "the majority of the masks furnished by the Red Cross (in California), which probably made up the bulk of those used, were undeniably too light and coarse in texture to do more than afford a comfortable feeling of safety on the part of the wearer." See Kellogg, 13.

populace on the whole was apparently not convinced of the need. Indeed, an editorial in the *San Diego Union* made obvious fun of the practice despite the serious intention of city health officer, Dr. E. P. Chartres-Martin:

> Modern civilization has abolished the mask as a part of human wearing apparel. . . only highwaymen, burglars, and hold-up men wear masks professionally. . . If the wearing of masks in the present emergency were a patriotic duty, we should certainly suggest red, white, and blue. . . We sincerely regret. . . that some of the younger women in public employment are compelled to wear these masks. We miss the pretty faces, and we have not yet learned to interpret the glances of the eyes that flash and sparkle above the concealing gauze. Finally, we would like to ask Dr. Chartres-Martin. . . if his orders extend to the billing and cooing of courting turtle doves?[13]

It is impossible to determine conclusively what, if any, effect the nasal spray, gauze masks, and closure of public facilities had on the spread of influenza. However, the foremost scholar of the epidemic argues that "the case and death rates of communities which had 'strict' closing orders were no better and often worse than elsewhere" and that "the influenza virus itself is (as we now know) so infinitely tiny that it can pass through any cloth, no matter how tightly woven."[14] As the incidence and seriousness of the epidemic began to subside, the City Board of Health decided to lift the existing quarantine on public entertainments and gatherings as of November 17. Schools were to remain closed for another two weeks as a necessary precaution. Camp Kearny also relaxed its strict quarantine by allowing liberty leaves in San Diego for officers and enlisted men.[15]

Then, in late November, the situation worsened. One hundred new cases of influenza were reported on November 29 with eight deaths within a two-day period. The disease spread to uptown residential districts from the waterfront and Hispanic quarter where it had previously been confined. An emergency isolation hospital for flu cases was readied in the office building

---

[13] *San Diego Union*, Oct. 21, 1918.

[14] Crosby, 74, 101.

[15] *San Diego Union*, Nov. 10, 14, 16, 1918.

of the old Mission brewery, just as the Fremont school had been similarly converted earlier. Faced with a new crisis, the City Board of Health decided to reimpose the previous quarantine on selected public facilities. However, the decision was not welcomed by all.[16] Claiming discrimination, theater managers refused to close their doors:

> If it is determined that any quarantine is necessary we favor one that will bring results and not the half-baked, wishy-washy closing order under which we operated for five weeks to the detriment of the entire community. The fact that the five weeks of closed amusements did not accomplish results spoke for itself. Why, then, if we would be consistent, do we not close all places where people gather?[17]

Other critics questioned the legal authority of the health board to enforce its ruling without the approval of the city council, while some owners of public accommodations feared a substantial loss of business. Mayor Louis Wilde, perhaps best known for defeating businessman and civic leader George Marston in the hotly contested "Geraniums vs. Smokestacks" mayoralty campaign of 1917 regarding San Diego's industrial development, addressed the economic issue in his endorsement of the quarantine:

> There is a class of people blind and indifferent to the death and sick rate, apparently unconcerned about everything else but nickel nursing and sight-seeing. If we cannot put life and health above dollars and pleasure for a few days we had better abolish the Bible and Constitution. I cannot see a particle of difference between the invasion of France by the heartless, lustful Huns and the invasion of our homes by some epidemic permitted by greed and politics.[18]

The city council apparently was unmoved by the mayor's claim that the influenza epidemic was the moral equivalent of war. The council refused to act on the board of health's ruling, although 165 new cases of the flu with

---

[16] *Ibid.*, Nov. 26, 28, 30; Dec. 1, 1918.

[17] *Ibid.*, Dec. 1, 1918.

[18] *Ibid.*, Dec. 2, 1918. For an analysis of the 1917 mayoralty campaign, see Uldis Ports, "Geraniums vs. Smokestacks: San Diego's Mayoralty Campaign of 1917," *Journal of San Diego History*, 21 (Summer, 1975), 50-56.

six deaths were reported for December 4. Such indecision prompted state intervention upon appeal from the city health authorities. On December 4, the State Board of Health ordered a quarantine of theaters, churches, schools, and other public places and gatherings in San Diego. Belatedly, on December 6, the city council endorsed this action and extended the quarantine to all places of business. The new, more inclusive quarantine only exempted businesses providing essential services from closure, such as banks, drug stores, grocery stores, meat markets, and the like. In addition, those employed in businesses which remained open and their customers were required by law to wear protective masks. Although those affected for the most part cooperated, some arrests were made when business personnel failed to comply with the ordinance.[19]

On December 9, the city council adopted a different approach to public health protection. The general quarantine was rescinded after only three days, but all persons were henceforth required to wear gauze masks, except in their homes. This method had been tried with apparent success in San Francisco and it generally won acceptance from San Diego businessmen and the public, especially during the Christmas shopping season. Yet, some ridiculed the practice by cutting holes in their masks to smoke cigars and cigarettes. Women occasionally wore theirs as harem-like veils, dangling loose over the chin. A few cynics fashioned masks with an extended snout resembling that of a pig. Nonetheless, after the implementation of the universal mask order, new flu cases began a steady decline. Seventy-six cases were reported on December 13, followed by 47 on December 14, and only 13 on December 15. The daily incidence of influenza continued to subside. On Christmas eve, the city council therefore discontinued the compulsory wearing of masks. Schools remained closed until January 6, 1919.[20]

---

[19] *San Diego Union*, Dec. 4-7, 9, 1918.

[20] *Ibid.*, Dec. 10-12, 15-16, 14, 1918; Jan. 2, 6, 1919. In a letter to *Ibid.*, Jan. 2, 1919, Wilbur F. Gearhart contended that the face mask induced shallow breathing and thus respiratory diseases. He asserted: "The contention that the wearing of flu' masks has caused the cessation of epidemics in certain places, is about as tenable as the theory that a dog barking at the moon causes the latter, out of fear, to disappear behind a cloud." Violations of San Diego's mask ordinance are discussed briefly in Richard Crawford, "The Past Comes Alive," *History News*,

Table 8.1

Births, Deaths, and Rates for 1918

Births:	1,559	Rate per 1000:	16.27
Deaths:	1,667*	Rate per 1000:	18.12

*Due to Flu: 30.46% (Public Health Records that would allow a breakdown by age are missing.)

Source: *Annual Report of the Department of Public Health*, City of San Diego, 1920.

Although not at an alarming daily rate, new influenza cases lingered on in San Diego until the winter of 1919. However, the situation was much worse in cities to the north. The early months of the year saw a disturbing rise in the incidence of the disease in San Francisco and Los Angeles. In the latter, which refused to impose a universal mask ordinance, an organization was formed to care for "flu orphans," left destitute by the death of their parents. For January 11, Los Angeles reported 715 new cases and 22 deaths. Los Angeles deaths registered as due to influenza and pneumonia were 178 and 177 for the weeks ending, respectively, on January 18 and January 25. These were the highest mortality figures since mid November of the previous year. Such statistics caused grave concern in San Diego since it was alleged that infected individuals traveling south had reinfected members of the local community at time when the San Diego epidemic was waning.[21]

The local board of health urged San Diegans not to go to Los Angeles and other cities to the north unless on the most pressing business. On January 14, authorities at Camp Kearny declared Los Angeles "off limits" for members of the 16th Army Division. This quarantine lasted until February 7, 1919. Although local health officials debated a similar action against Los

---

San Diego Historical Society, 21 (Feb. 1985), 2. For a discussion of San Francisco's experience with a comparable universal mask ordinance, see Crosby, 101-116.

[21]*San Diego Union*, Jan. 10-11, 1919. Statistics on San Francisco's weekly rate of influenza cases and weekly influenza and pneumonia deaths in San Francisco and Los Angeles are available in Crosby, 60-61, 114.

Angeles, nothing was done.[22] However, the *San Diego Union* kept the issue alive in several editorials, including the one excerpted below:

> Whatever else the health authorities of Los Angeles are doing in their efforts to stay the progress of this disease, it is certain that they neither insist on the wearing of masks nor discourage citizens from leaving the city. Many of these persons come to San Diego, where we have almost stayed the progress of the ailment. Some of our health authorities are of the opinion that if it were not for this Los Angeles immigration this city would be practically free of the influenza germ.[23] As the epidemic began to ease in the state by the early Spring, such allegations were no longer newsworthy. In the meantime, Spanish influenza had become not only a national crisis but a source of inter-city conflict.[24]

Throughout 1918, there were 4,392 cases and 324 deaths in San Diego. For 1919, the city reported 648 cases and 44 deaths. However, the worst was over by the end of 1918. About 7% of the San Diego population caught the flu from 1918 through 1919. The rate of infection, despite the concern and controversy it generated, was well below the national and worldwide average. However, the death of approximately 7% of those afflicted was comparable to San Francisco's flu mortality rate between September 1918 and January 1919 inclusive. San Francisco had the most severe influenza epidemic of any West Coast city. About 10% of the 550,000 residents caught the virus which came in two waves.[25]

Despite some similarity with San Francisco, the epidemic in San Diego was relatively mild when compared to large eastern cities like Boston, New York, and Philadelphia. In the latter, the mortality rate for one week in the critical month of October 1918 was 700 times the normal rate for influenza and pneumonia and for the entire epidemic period, 752.1 times the

---

[22] *San Diego Union*, Jan. 10-11, 14; Feb. 7, 1919.

[23] *Ibid.*, Jan. 20, 1919.

[24] *Ibid.*, Feb. 1, 13, 1919.

[25] The San Diego statistics can be found in Pourade, 5: 231. For San Francisco's statistics, see Crosby, 70, 91, 113-14; and Arseny K. Hernoff, "The Influenza Epidemic of 1918-1919 in San Francisco," *Military Surgeon*, 89 (Nov. 1941), 806-07.

usual rate. This forced the deceased to be gathered in carts as during Europe's bubonic plague or Black Death epidemic from 1347 to 1350.[26] Although many cities and towns in the country suffered from the flu, San Diego may have been spared the more serious consequences that hit some eastern cities because it was comparatively small, far from the war zone, and not at this time a major military staging area or important naval port. In addition, the protective measures imposed by the local health board and city government perhaps deserve some credit for containing the spread of infection. However, Kansas City, Missouri, which did not take such precautions as closing public amusements, was no harder hit than cities that took extreme measures.[27] In any event, with the possible exception of the "Hong Kong Flu" epidemics of 1957 and 1968-69, San Diego and the rest of the country would not experience an influenza scare that was even remotely similar until the much milder swine flu panic of the mid 1970s. Investigators then suspected that this strain was related to the one that caused the great epidemic of 1918-19.[28]

In retrospect, as with the swine flu, scientists were unable to develop a safe and effective vaccine for Spanish influenza, although useless ones were tried. Under such conditions, quackery flourished in San Diego and elsewhere. Various advertised potions promised an effective preventive or miracle cure. The lack of understanding regarding the causes of the killer virus was reflected in such locally recommended treatments as spraying the nose and throat, seeking high altitudes, or getting outdoor exercise. A Boston physician, Dr. Charles E. Page, suggested that excessive clothing

---

[26]Persico, 80, 84. For the number of deaths due to influenza and pneumonia in major American cities, see Crosby, 60-61. Statistics were unavailable for San Diego, but San Francisco had an excess death rate from influenza and pneumonia during the epidemic of 669.4. For such statistics on major cities, including Philadelphia, see unnumbered pages between 207 and 217 in Crosby.

[27]Persico, 31.

[28]For evidence of a possible link between Spanish influenza and swine flu, see J. Donald Millar and June E. Osborn, "Precursors of the Scientific Decision-Making process Leading to the 1976 national Immunization Campaign," in June E. Osborn (ed.), *Influenza In America* (New York, 1977), 16; and Crosby, 218-19, 298-306. See also Collier, 306-308.

caused the flu. In Chicago, people were advised to chew food carefully, avoid tight clothes, tight shoes, and tight gloves. An Oklahoma doctor, Alexander Leeds, recommended pulling out teeth and tonsils to cure people of the flu.[29] Even Surgeon General Rupert Blue of the U.S. Public Health Service could do little more than caution people to "cover up each cough and sneeze; if you don't you'll spread disease."[30] In San Diego, the late Grace Kauber was the mother of two small children ill with influenza in 1918. Her prescription for recovery required extensive rest. She remembers "that several young people died because they got out of bed too soon. It took a great deal of care to get over the flu then." She did not let her 4-year-old son Philip and 6-year-old daughter Alice "get up at all until I was absolutely sure their temperatures were back to normal."[31]

At present, Spanish influenza is still a medical mystery. Little is known about its causes, why it disappeared shortly after the war despite the recurrence of a milder epidemic in early 1920, and why it was disproportionately fatal to adults between the ages of 20 and 40, when influenza historically had its most lethal impact on the very young and especially the elderly.[32] Perhaps the causal explanation of a popular rhyme of the era, which tried to inject humor into an otherwise tragic situation, is as revealing as any: "I had a little bird and its name was Enza. I opened the window and in-flew-Enza." It was not until 1933, when the virus that causes influenza was isolated under an electron microscope, that more scientific explanations could be offered for a disease whose many mutations

---

[29]Hoehling, 101-02; and Persico, 31.

[30]*New York Times*, Sept. 21, 1918. For an evaluation of various methods used to combat the epidemic in California and the nation, see Kellogg, 4-23.

[31]As quoted in Lew Scarr, "In 1918 the flu wasn't inconvenient, it was deadly," *San Diego Union*, Mar. 10, 1985.

[32]See graphs of comparative influenza death rates by age groups in Alfred Crosby, Jr., "The Influenza Pandemic of 1918," in Osborn, 6. Also, see *Epidemic and Peace*, 203-04, 215-23.

challenged the medical community.[33] One of these mutations, the Spanish strain of 1918-19, was fatal to more humans than any other disease in a period of similar duration in world history. The Plague of Justinian, beginning in 542 A.D., reportedly killed 100 million people, but it lasted 50 years. It took three years for the bubonic Black Death to wipe out one-third of Europe's population. Spanish influenza had worked its devastating will over mankind in about four months.[34] Given its swift, sudden impact, had the virulent pandemic continued on an accelerated course, much of the human race would conceivably have been eliminated. Thus, even in this fearful age of potential nuclear holocaust, one is reminded of T. S. Eliot's hauntingly poetic prophesy that the world will end "not with a bang, but a whimper."[35]

Perhaps a final irony regarding the epidemic in San Diego and southern California is the fact that the general area had been highly touted in the late nineteenth century for its restorative powers of climate, which prompted a substantial health rush between 1870 and 1900. Indeed, Dr. Peter C. Remondino's book, *The Mediterranean Shores of America: Southern California, Its Climate, Physical, and Meteorological Conditions*, published in 1892, promoted the migration of health seekers, hoping to cure pulmonary and respiratory ailments in particular.[36] However, even allegedly healthful

---

[33]The jingle is related in Luckingham, 3. A discussion of the scientific quest for the causes and cure of influenza can be found in Hoehling, 193-99; Persico, 84, 86; Crosby, *Epidemic and Peace*, 264-306; and Pettit, 12-49.

[34]Crosby, *Epidemic and Peace*, 215; and Collier, 306. Useful works on the bubonic plague include William M. Bowsky, ed., *The Black Death: A Turning Point in History?* (New York, 1970); and Robert S. Gottfried, *The Black Death: Natural and Human Disaster in Medieval Europe* (New York, 1983).

[35]For an analysis of "The Hollow Men," the poem from which the quotation is taken, see George Williamson, *A Reader's Guide to T.S. Eliot: A Poem-by-Poem Analysis* (New York, 1966), 154-62.

[36]See John E. Baur, *The Health Seekers of Southern California, 1870-1900* (San Marino, CA: 1959), 10-12. For evidence of the development of a health legend in San Diego, also see Billy M. Jones, *Health-Seekers in the Southwest, 1817-1900* (Norman, OK, 1967), 83, 87, 102, and 153. Remondino, who moved to San Diego in 1873 for his health, established the city's initial private hospital and in 1875 was appointed City Physician. He also served as president of the County Board of Health, president of the San Diego County and Southern California Medical

Southern California was not immune from the world-wide impact of the flu epidemic. This may explain why there is apparently no evidence of former "health boosters" attempting to reconcile the health-giving properties of the region with the obvious devastation caused by influenza. The pandemic was simply too powerful and perhaps too embarrassing to easily explain away, especially in a celebrated health-seekers' paradise.

Society, and vice president of the California Medical Society. Later, this former "health booster" was officially active in San Diego's fight against the influenza outbreak. For a brief sketch of his career, see "Research Archives features exhibit on early San Diego physician," *History News* San Diego Historical Society, 21 (Feb. 1985), 3. Remondino's collected papers are contained in seven boxes at the San Diego Historical Society.

Chapter 9: Guatemala City

David McCreery

The months from the end of 1917 to early 1919 were difficult ones for Guatemala and must have led many of the the republic's inhabitants to ponder Job's fate. Beginning on Christmas Eve, 1917, with a severe earthquake, a succession of natural disasters wracked the country, laying waste to the capital and killing tens of thousands of people in the towns and countryside. The government's inability to respond effectively to these calamities not only aggravated the population's suffering but threw into stark relief the political and economic exhaustion of the existing regime, helping pave the way for the overthrow of the dictator in 1920. The most deadly of the year's afflictions, the world-wide influenza pandemic of 1918-1919, which appeared in Guatemala in August-September, 1918, and lasted until March of the following year. This chapter examines the course of the epidemic in that country, and, particularly, in Guatemala City,[1] the efforts of public agencies and private groups to deal with the disease, and short and long term effects on Guatemala of the influenza outbreak.

On the night of December 25, 1917, and continuing intermittently for several weeks thereafter, earthquakes, the worst in the history of the capital, rocked Guatemala City and leveled most structures. Recovery was slow. A

---

[1]An unpublished census taken in 1914 recorded the population of guatemala as 2,183,166 and Guatemala City as 99,099: U.S. Department of State, "Documents relating to the internal affairs of Guatemala, 1910-1929, microfilm, roll #20.

report issued a year later by the Ministry of the Interior [Gobernación] indicated:

> The National Palace, the theaters, the asylums, private houses, the hospitals, cemeteries, barracks, schools, libraries, museums, the aqueducts [which brought in the city's water], the churches, . . . were totally destroyed or severely damaged. . . . The parks, plazas, the patios of the public buildings and the open spaces around the city. . .served and serve as refuge for many of the inhabitants, who suffered and suffer with resignation their fate."[2]

Beyond shooting a few looters as exemplary punishment, patching up the aqueducts, and burning the corpses exposed in the cemeteries, the government did little to meet the problems resulting from the earthquakes. The dictator Manuel Estrada Cabrera, in power since the assassination of his predecessor in 1898, had almost entirely retreated to his estate of La Palma on the outskirts of the capital and, in paranoid if justified fear of his many enemies, rarely appeared in public. He ruled by confusion, treachery, and inaction.[3] Not until February did a *Comité General de Auxiliar de Guatemala*, made of of "leading citizens," organize the clean up and drainage of the refugee camps, and only in April did a modest government sanitary service begin to proffer daily medical inspections. But, ominously, when the rainy season began again in May,[4] few of the refugees had been able to leave the camps, and most of the public buildings, including the hospitals, were yet to be rebuilt or adequately repaired. Much of the population entered the

---

[2]Ministerio de Gobernación, *Memoria-1918* (Guatemala City, 1918), 5ff; see also *Diario de Centro América* (Guatemala City) [the *Diario* is the major newspaper of the city], Nov. 17, Dec. 7, 1917, Jan. 1, 1920; and the *Imparcia* (Guatemala City), Dec. 24, 1937. Professor L. Feldman has completed a catalogue of earthquakes in Central America and is at work on a full length study of that of 1917-18.

[3]Estrada Cabrere's rule is the subject of Miguel Angel Asturias' famous novel *El Señor Presidente*, trans. by Frances Partridge (New York, 1982).

[4]Guatemala City normally has a "rainy season from late April until October, with almost daily showers, and a "dry season," when it rarely rains, from October to April. Because of the predominance of weathered, volcanic soil around the capital, the countryside tended to alternate mud with dust.

rains of the *invierno* ("winter") huddled together in tents and makeshift housing without adequate sanitation or medical facilities.

The *Diario de Centro América*[5] remarked in June, 1918,[6] and without naming the disease, on a "great epidemic" in Spain, but there was no public mention of an epidemic or of influenza in Guatemala until late October. In fact, however, the disease had arrived more than two months earlier. The *Ministerio de Gobernación* began collecting, but not publishing, statistics on influenza deaths as early as September 2,[7] suggesting that the disease must already have been present in the country for at least a week or two. Perhaps the government discouraged prior comment on the pandemic in the hopes, shared by many towns and nations in these months,[8] that a serious plague would pass Guatemala by. Public health conditions among the poor were generally so bad that a disease, unless and until it reached epidemic proportions, would have occasioned little notice or comment, and the press was unlikely to have paid influenza much attention until it appeared to threaten the "better classes" or the rural labor supply. For the tiny and tightly knit elite of the capital, local events reported in the newspapers were, in any event, already old news. Not until October 22[9] did the *Diario* confess that the "influenza epidemic is universal," attacking residents of the capital and the departments.[10] But the disease did not yet seem a serious danger.

---

[5]The *Diario de Centro América* was the only newspaper, other than the government paper of record, the *Guatemalteco* (Guatemala City), consistently available for these months.

[6]*Diario de Centro América*, June 3, 11, 1918.

[7]Archivo General de Centro América (Hereafter A.G.C.A.), uncatalogued papers of the Ministerio de Gobernación, *legajo* (bundle) #29399. Only the figures beginning Dec. 1, 1918, were published: *Diario de Centro América*, Jan. 10, 1919.

[8]On public reaction to flu in towns which shared many similarities with Guatemala City, see Bradford Luckingham, *Epidemic in the Southwest, 1918-1919* (El Paso, 1984).

[9]*Diario de Centro América* Oct. 22, 1918.

[10]Based on the French system, Guatemala was divided into some twenty-two departments rather than states or provinces. Apparently, Guatemala had had serious influenza epidemics in 1867, 1870, and 1890 but had kept no statistics: *Diario de Centro América*, Jan. 10, 1919.

Indeed, the unpublished government figures show influenza declining in the capital from October to November.[11]

The epidemic appears to have entered Guatemala more or less simultaneously from Mexico to the west and from the Caribbean to the north, along the rail line from Puerto Barrios.[12] Perhaps because it traveled by rail rather than foot, the virus, except for a few isolated and mild cases, initially leap-frogged the north and did not reappear there in a serious form until several months later. It took quick and vigorous root in the western highlands, however, from San Marcos on the Mexican border to Chimaltenango, just a few miles northwest of Guatemala City. Weeks before the capital admitted to serious difficulties, the governor of San Marcos issued public instructions on battling influenza:

TO THE PEOPLE

If you are indisposed, with chills, pain in the bones, headache, fever, sore throat: these are the symptoms of INFLUENZA.
It is necessary to lie down.

***

One must cover oneself without an excess of clothing and keep the room well ventilated.
It is necessary to drink milk, gruel, barley water, etc. Abstain from meat, wine, beer and other spirituous drinks. You ought not to go out except in cases of absolute necessity; avoid walking a lot or with your feet uncovered....

***

You ought not to cough or sneeze in the presence of others, for if you do infection is certain.

***

Do not go to wakes.
Do not sweep without dampening the floor.

---

[11]A.G.C.A., Gobernación, legajo 29399.

[12]*Diario de Centro América*, Oct. 22, Nov. 12, 16, 1918.

Do not use irritating disinfectants such as sulfur, etc. Instead, burn the fruit and leaves of the eucalyptus.[13]

On November 30, the government sent two doctors to Chimaltenango to check on the situation there. They encountered a preview of what lay in store for Guatemala City. The epidemic, the doctors reported, was a "common" influenza but with characteristics of the Spanish strain: "quick onset, very strong headache, pains in the body, high temperature and nausea. . .; the following day congestion begins and bronchial-pneumonia may attack. . . with blood-specked mucous, etc."[14] Half the population had fallen ill, but, the doctors felt, much of the blame lay with the *indio* victims themselves for their "miserable hygiene:" Most of the sick sleep on the ground;

> when the illness hits them, they get drunk, and the terrible cold of morning finds them, sweating and lying in soaked clothing on the damp soil....The next day they get up repeatedly in temperatures of 39 degrees to go to the toilet. Is it any wonder they get pneumonia?

On the other hand, the *ladinos*[15] who, according to the visiting doctors, recovered more quickly from the effects of the influenza than did the *indio*s showed no interest in assisting their stricken neighbors: "Their only concern is to get back to business as quickly as possible." It was clear that those who came down with the influenza had less need of doctors than of relatives, friends, or nurses to care from them. But in many cases entire families found themselves "with no one to bring them water or food, let alone medicine."

On December 11 the *chapines* (residents of the capital) finally awoke to the disaster in their midst. It was now clear, the *Diario de Centro América*

---

[13]A.G.C.A., Ministerio de Gobernación, legajo 28399.

[14]Ministerio de Gobernación, *Memoria-1919* (Guatemala City, 1919), 53ff.

[15]In Guatemala the *ladino* is an individual of "European" or "national" habits and dress who speaks Spanish. "*Indio*" and "*ladino*" are not racial terms.

admitted, that "many" cases of Spanish influenza existed in the capital.[16] the government would have to take action. In a long piece, "The Sanitary Question," the paper outlined what it considered to be the necessary steps. Because, it said, epidemics were propagated by dirt and by close conditions, the authorities should close all schools, churches, taverns, bordellos, and similar establishments and forbid all gatherings, processions, wakes, and the like. They must initiate a general clean up, removing trash from the streets and making certain that sanitary conditions existed in the camps, in the central market, and among street vendors of food and sweets. Medicines should be made available to the ill as needed, not sold by corrupt officials. The situation in the capital was particularly dangerous because of

> [t]he conditions in which the city has remained after the earthquake, the heaping together of the inhabitants in the camps and emergency tents, the lack of drains in some areas, the indifference in which a painful struggle for life leaves the poor and the indolence and ignorance of the most elemental measures of hygiene among even many of the better off.[17]

What was needed was "water, water, and more water," both for a general clean up and to dampen down the dust which, with Guatemala's volcanic soil, quickly followed the end of the rainy season.[18] Masks would be a good idea. On the 13th the *Diario* returned to the idea of masks, and on the 14th called for the systematic watering of the many unpaved streets in the capital. It also began to publish, at regular intervals, and set apart in blocks, admonitions on how to avoid the influenza:

> Be careful with the cold. Protect the chest, throat and lungs. Don't go without sleep. Don't go out at night. Remember that most deaths result of not taking care of oneself, either because they had to go out late at night to get medicine or because with a cold and a small fever they went to a party. Use an overcoat

---

[16]*Diario de Centro América*, Dec. 11, 1918.

[17]*Ibid.*, Jan. 20, 1919.

[18]This version is from *Ibid*.

> and a mask. Don't catch cold. Influenza is only deadly to those who don't take care of themselves.[19]

In a series of recommendations which would, no doubt, have been a great help to the city's poor had they been able to afford a newspaper or been able to read it, the *Diario* suggested: "Wash the rooms with water boiled with eucalyptus leaves. Don't let many people sleep in the same room, and don't worry yourself[!]."19 Newspaper advertisements for patent medicines guaranteed to cure influenza multiplied.[20]

The *Diario* was not alone in offering ideas on how to meet the epidemic. The *Consejo Superior de Salubridad* (National Health Council), set up originally to fight malaria and yellow fever and headed up by the local representative of the Rockefeller Foundation suggested:

> 1) Quarantining all infected parts of the country.
>
> 2) Prohibiting all public meetings involving ten or more persons.
>
> 3) Isolating all those ill and requiring them to rest in bed.
>
> 4) Prohibiting spitting in public.
>
> 5) Instructing public to use handkerchief when coughing or sneezing in public.
>
> 6) Requiring that all secretions relevant to influenza be burned.
>
> 7) Making masks mandatory.
>
> 8) Vaccinating the population.[21]

---

[19] *Ibid.*, Jan. 7, 1919.

[20] See, for example, *Ibid.*, Dec. 18, 1918.

[21] *Ibid.*, Dec. 14, 1918.

The city council of the capital petitioned the governor to order the closing of all public gathering places,[22] and on the 16th he complied.[23] The *Diario* kept up its campaign in favor of water.[24]

On the 17th the *Diario* called a meeting of the capital's doctors in order to discuss what should be done to combat the epidemic. Only a few, the paper subsequently complained, showed up, and they wasted much time in pointlessly debating whether the disease presently attacking the city was an "influenza" or a "grippe" and in congratulating themselves that its presence was less severe in Guatemala City than elsewhere. They did agree, however, that while there seemed to be no specific or effective remedies for influenza, masks could be useful to slow its propagation, especially among the--presumably more disease-ridden--*indios*. Convalescence was very important. After hearing descriptions of the walls along the streets of Chimaltenango made "red with the bloody mucous" spit up by suffers, the doctors recommended placing boxes of sawdust on street corners to serve as spittoons.[25] The also suggested issuing a pamphlet outlining preventive measures and remedies.

The same day that the doctors met at the behest of the *Diario*, President Estrada Cabrera, in an evident confession of the state's inability to deal with the emergency, called together members of the local elite at his retreat La Palma. He asked them to create an *Asociación Nacional de Salubridad* (National Health Association) to organize the campaign against the pandemic. Quickly constituted, the *Asociación*, in turn, telegraphed the departmental governors calling on them to set up similar local associations and issued, with the governor of the department of Guatemala, emergency regulations:

---

[22]*Ibid.*

[23]*Ibid.*, Dec. 17, 1917.

[24]*Ibid.*, Jan. 17, 1918.

[25]The *cacos* (bums) of the streets quickly took to stealing these and selling them, often to merchants in the central market for food storage. *Ibid.*, Dec. 26, 1918.

1) Use of the mask was obligatory;

2) Everyone was to water down the street in front of their house twice a day;

3) Half the pharmacies in the city were to be open at any time, round the clock;

4) All food sold on the streets must be adequately protected against dust;

5) All meeting places were to be closed and meetings prohibited.[26]

They set up a Sanitary Police and ordered it to enforce the new meeting and mask regulations, to take the ill to hospital or to dispose of the bodies, to make sure trash was picked up, and to carry out disinfections where needed.[27] President Estrada Cabrera promised 500,000 pesos for the group's activities.[28]

For the purposes of fighting the epidemic, the *Asociación* divided Guatemala City into eight *cantones* (districts) and appointed and paid doctors and doctors' assistants for each. It set up an Office of Immediate Assistance to which the worst cases were to be dispatched. As the more candid of the leaders of the *Asociación* themselves admitted, however, "doctors don't matter much. . . . What is really necessary are a sufficient number of nurses."[29] To this end they organized a corps of paid nurses under the volunteer direction of a wife and a daughter of local elites. Women "of all conditions" enrolled. The directors initially admitted individuals on the basis of two recommendations, but they soon discovered, or so it was claimed, that men were "very accommodating" and gave recommendations too easily to women of "doubtful character;" they decided henceforth to

---

[26]*Ibid.*, Dec. 19, 1918. These regulations the government subsequently extended to the entire country.

[27]*Ibid.*, Dec. 24, 1918; Gobernación, *Memoria-1919*, 89.

[28]*Diario de Centro América*, Dec. 19, 1918. In 1918 40 pesos equaled approximately one U.S. dollar.

[29]Gobernación, *Memoria-1919*, 55.

accept only letters from *Señoras* (married women)! The heads of the nurse corps noted, though, that if many of of the women allowed to join in the first rush had pursued "immoral and irregular" lives before, they served very satisfactorily in their new calling; at least one of these, the patients agreed, was an "angel." "[I]f some poor women led a life of which society disapproves," they suggested, in a sentiment with which North American Progressives of the era would have agreed, "it was, in the first instance, because they lacked an opportunity to work at a decent occupation."[30] Some eighty women of all social backgrounds worked as nurses during the epidemic, most laboring in the poorer parts of town and the tent camps. How many, if any, died, is not known.

The civilian population complained repeatedly of the "filthy" condition of soldiers and protested that their barracks, located usually in the center of town, served to propagate the epidemic. The residents of San Marcos city, for example, pointed out that some of the troops there had not bathed in a year![31] In the *Cuartel de Artillería of Quezaltenango* hygiene was "*palabra muerta*" (a dead word).[32] Local residents blamed regular troops, too, for spreading influenza as the government shifted them about the country. Soldiers, the newspaper reported, deserted by pretending to die of flu and then paying off the grave diggers![33] The army countered this sort of news and accusation with the unlikely boast that the barracks had suffered not a single case of flu. The health conditions of and for the soldiers, the commanders claimed, could not be improved.[34]

The influenza pandemic largely ran its course in Guatemala city between October, 1918, and early February, 1919.

---

[30] *Ibid.*, 22-3, 84-5.

[31] *Diario de Centro América*, Nov. 16, 1918.

[32] *Ibid.*, Jan. 16, 1919.

[33] *Ibid.*, Jan. 28, 1919.

[34] *Ibid.*, Jan. 13, 1919.

Table 9.1

Number of Deaths--Guatemala City

Month	*All*	*Flu*	*Month*	*All*	*Flu*
1918					
January	208		July	306	
February	150		August	329	
March	164		September	252	26
April	198		October	390	158
May	204		November	235	50
June	259		December	712	459
			1919		
			January*		274*

(*January figures are incomplete.)

Source: Archivo General de Centro América, Gobernación, Legajo 29399 and 29402.

As early as December 30 various doctors in the capital claimed to see the epidemic in retreat,[35] and the peak day for deaths seems to have been January 5, 1919, with 32.[36]

While the influenza raged through the camps and the saloons of Guatemala City, the *Diario* was clearly more preoccupied with conditions in the countryside, and particularly those on the coffee plantations (*fincas*). Coffee prices, after the vicissitudes resulting from the recent war, were good, but the harvest would rot unpicked unless labor could be had.[37] And the epidemic had hit at the peak of the harvest season. The paper each day reported horrors from the *fincas*: on Mirandilla the owner was ill and had lost half the harvest because the workers were either sick or had run away; at La Providencia in Palo Gordo, a wife died, leaving a sick husband and child and all of the workers ill; the epidemic decimated the population of the *fincas* around Patulul and on the south coast: on some plantations 50% to 60% of the workers had died. The harvest was "paralyzed" in Barbarena and

---

[35]*Ibid.*, Dec. 30, 1918.

[36]A.G.C.A., Gobernación, legajo 29399.

[37]*Diario de Centro América*, Dec. 20, 1918.

"Suspended" at Pochuta, and *fincas* had lost 80% of their harvest.[38] On Nueva California the administrator overwhelmed the *mozos* with a variety of herbal teas, as well as "*sulfato de quina, aspirina, ipecacuana, Laudano de Sydenham, polvos de Dower, calomel, purgantes salinas, sulfatos de calcio, acido fénico y profilácticos y curativos por la via tintura de yoda*!"[39] Many more workers would have succumbed to influenza, the *Diario* suggested, "but for the heroic and unequal struggle [of plantation owners and administrators] in which silent love and altruism triumphed."[40] All but a few skeptics[41] predicted a severe blow to the economy resulting from the shortfall in available laborers.

Whereas the influenza, according to the newspaper, "[did] not kill more than 5% to 10% of the [urban] population,"[42] its impact on the rural *indios* of the western highlands appears to have been much more severe;[43] they were "dying like flies."[44] It is only possible to say "appears," however, because an oppressed and illiterate population ignored by the state, except as a source of cheap labor, leaves few and inadequate records. The *ladinos* of the capital tended to see the *indios*' problem as one of living conditions and behavior: "The mortality here is numerous among the *indios* who live in shacks poorly roofed, packed together, piled three or four in the same bed on the ground and surrounded by the mucous they have spit up. . . . All of this, together with the vicious customs so rooted in the *indio* class have been factors very useful in the propagation of the disease."[45] Such conditions

---

[38]*Ibid.*, Dec. 20-21, 23, 26, 1918, Jan. 14, 16, 22, 1919.

[39]*Ibid.*, Jan. 28, 1919.

[40]*Ibid.*

[41]See, for example, *Ibid.*, Feb. 4, 1919.

[42]*Ibid.*, Dec. 27, 1918.

[43]Compare Alfred W. Crosby, *Epidemic and Peace 1918* (Westport, CT, 1976), chap. 12 "Samoa and Alaska."

[44]*Diario de Centro América*, Dec. 17, 1918.

[45]Gobernación, *Memoria-1919*, 57-8.

probably aggravated the epidemic's impacts--and state officials did not help the situation by bringing gangs of *indios* from outlying villages into the towns to clean up trash[46]--but inadequate nutrition, endemic disease, and parasites brought on at least in part by the forced labor and the land losses attendant on the recent expansion of coffee export production[47] weakened the population and left many of them especially susceptible to the influenza. The disease among *indios* more commonly, or so doctors reported,[48] took the form of pneumonia and hemorrhages than was the case with *ladinos*. Those who fell ill could rarely afford or have access to a doctor, but turned, instead, to the *brujo* or *curandero* (the "witch doctor" or the "medicine man"). Given what medical doctors could do for flu victims, treatment by the *brujo* and, more importantly, the family, was probably at least as effective. In many areas of the highlands the indigenous population had successfully resisted Spanish and national patterns of concentration and continued to live dispersed in the *monte* (countryside) and in tiny hamlets. Others fled the larger villages for the open areas at the onset of the epidemic. There death found them, and whole families succumbed, to be buried without markers or eaten by animals and birds. The "army" of *indio* workers was being "decimated as a battalion cut down by enemy machine guns," the *Diario* protested, and government officials cared not at all, for they thought of "the *indio*. . .like the sheep, an eternal element."[49]

Influenza attacked the northwestern part of the country first, then the capital, and came to the northeast last of all. Western departments reported the disease in epidemic proportions by mid-October; the director of the San Marcos hospital remembered the two weeks of October 24-November 8 as

---

[46]*Diario de Centro América*, Dec. 28, 1918.

[47] See David McCreery, "An Odious Feudalism: Mandamientos and Commercial Agriculture in Guatemala, 1861-1920," *Latin American Perspectives*, 13 (Winter, 1983), 99-117.

[48]*Diario de Centro América*, Jan. 2, 1919.

[49]*Ibid.*, Dec. 27, 1918.

"horrible."[50] By the end of the year it was passing.[51] In contrast, the capital only took serious, if belated, notice of influenza in mid-December and the disease peaked in early and mid-January, 1919.

Table 9.2

"Worst Days" by Department

Suchitepéquez--Dec. 29	Retalhuleu--Jan. 19
Sololá--"end of December"	Progreso--Jan. 26
Totonicapan--Jan. 1	Zacapa--Jan. 27
Jalapa--Jan. 3	Petén--Jan. 27
Santa Rosa--Jan. 5	Amatitlán--Jan. 8
Huehuetenango--Jan. 6	Alta Verapaz--Feb. 3
Quiché--Jan. 12	Jutiapa--Jan. 16
Baja Verapaz--"at present" [early February]	

Source: *Diario de Centro América*, Jan. 29, Feb. 5, 1919.

---

[50]A.G.C.A., Gobernación, legajo 29406.

[51]See, for example, the end-of-the-year reports by the governors of Suchitepéquez and Quezaltenango in *Ibid.*, legajo 29402.

Table 9.3

Illness by Department

Department	Jan. 20	Jan. 31	Feb. 4	Feb. 12	Feb. 27	Mar. 9
Sacatepéques	517	183	146	64	6	--
Petén	12	0	--	87	--	--
Amatitlán	635	538	460	425	200	60
Huehuenan	12,400	--	5,100	3,000	1,412	1,186
Quiché	1,749	760	899	389	189	75
Retalhuleu	61	--	5	5	0	2
Progreso*	1,361	--	1,235	738	392	198
Jalapa*	9,223	1,523	1,657	902	144	82
Totonicapán	151	75	71	56	--	0
Zacapa*	579	1,079	--	1,195	538	134
Suchitepéquez	841	96	75	--	0	0
Escuintla	1,075	878	554	309	50	--
Chiquimula*	1,616	1,959	2,034	1,897	625	427
SanMarcos	--	--	--	0	--	--
BajaVerapaz*	2,658	2,415	2,046	--	682	249
AltaVerapaz*	2,788	--	2,064	988	1,780	643
Sololá	--	25	--	--	--	--
SantaRosa*	2,041	--	55	--	93	55
Jutiapa*	2,014	1,781	1,666	1,280	307	--
Quezaltenango	4,125	--	1,378	871	288	71
Chuimaltenango	--	--	--	--	--	--

(*--Departments of the North and East)

Source: *Diario de Centro América*, Jan. 21, Feb. 1, 5, 28, Mar. 10, 1919.

As late as January 3, the authorities at Cobán, the departmental capital of the Alta Verapaz, and at Zacapa, to the south, reported no evidence of the epidemic in the area.[52] The situation soon changed, however, and by the 10th, influenza cases in Cobán were growing at the rate of 10% a day.[53] On the 16th Chiquimula reported that the disease "had developed recently," and Morales (near the United Fruit Company headquarters of Bananera) noted that "only now has influenza arrived."[54] By the 18th it was sowing "panic" in Salamá. Deaths ran as high as 30 a day (in a

[52] *Diario de Centro América*, Jan. 3, 1918.

[53] *Ibid.*, Jan. 10, 1919.

[54] *Ibid.*, Jan. 16, 1919.

population of 15,000) and grave diggers could not keep up; bodies had to be dumped two or three to a grave.[55] The epidemic was still increasing in the Salamá, Rabinal, Cubulco, and Zacapa at the end of January and probably peaked in this area during early to mid-February, a month or more after the rest of the country. Scattered notes in March mention as many as 13 deaths in a single day around Cobán.

Influenza was no longer a major public health concern in the capital by the end of February. The newspaper and the *Asociación Nacional*, however, argued that preventive measures had to be continued, and they worried about a possible "second wave," as reported in parts of Europe and North America.[56] Unless the delayed outbreak in the northeast was a "second wave," or unless this phenomenon in Guatemala was so mild as to have been lost in the generally poor public health situation and faulty reporting, there was no "second wave." Or perhaps, given the high death rates for Guatemala City in October, followed by a decrease in November and then a rapid rise in December and January, the main attack in the capital was itself a "second wave." In any event, on February 15 headlines trumpeted "No Deaths [in Guatemala City] Yesterday as a Result of Flu," and on the 19th the paper reported no new cases of the disease in the capital.[57]

Table 9.4

Deaths in Guatemala City

February 5	3	February 18	0
February 13	4	February 20	3
February 14	0	February 26	0

Source: *Diario de Centro América*, Feb. 6, 14, 15, 19, 21, 27, 1919.

---

[55] *Ibid.*, Jan. 18, 1919.

[56] See, for example, comments in *Ibid.*, Jan. 21, 1919.

[57] *Ibid.*, Jan. 22, 28, Feb. 4, 11, 1919.

The *Asociación Nacional* began to wind down its activities. On January 25, they dismissed a third of the canton doctors and their assistants and on February 8 let the rest go, though they sent nine of these to aid work in the departments. On February they turned the duties of the Sanitary Police over to the regular police. In a final tally, the *Asociación* reported that it raised 950,077 pesos and spent 847,230, chiefly on salaries for the doctors, doctors assistants, and nurses. It had given out 5,904 tickets for free doctors' visits and 7,704 prescriptions for free medicine, and distributed 40,000 liters of soup, 445 shirts, as well as sheets and blankets, and 196 coffins. For the city, they estimated that 7,380[58] had come down with influenza, of whom 757 died, giving a morbidity (per 1000) of 74.5, a mortality of 7.6, and a case rate mortality of 102.5. Certainly this was an underestimate but probably more accurate than figures for the rest of the country. On March 7, the government lifted the ban on meetings and gatherings.[59]

It is useful, even given their evident imperfections to examine some of the broader statistics of the pandemic in Guatemala.

---

[58]*Ibid.*, Feb. 15, 19, 1919.

[59]See the final report in Gobernación, *Memoria-1919*, 64ff.

Table 9.5

Impact of Influenza by Department (per 1000)

Department	*Population*	*Morbidity*	*Mortality*	*Case Rate*
Guatemala	203,176	282	8.4	30
Quezaltegango*	185,112	81	23.0	284
Amatitlán	43,824	140	18.6	133
Alta Verapaz*	159,456	51	11.3	222
Baja Verapaz*	66,771	85	39.2	458
Chiquimula	111,487	68	8.0	117
Chimaltenango*	105,570	71	1.9	27
Escuintla	64,233	470	15.1	32
Huehuetenango*	179,886	220	33.8	153
Izabal	10,989	114	6.4	56
Jalapa	48,276	235	42.1	179
Jutiapa	88,290	161	18.3	114
Progreso	37,731	195	14.3	73
Petén	7,317	70	2.6	37
Quiché*	150,931	206	38.9	184
Retalhuleu	41,910	27	5.3	199
Sololá*	117,774	198	40.8	206
Sacatepéquez	51,192	92	20.2	219
Suchitepéquez	74,217	63	18.8	300
Santa Rosa	96,255	187	34.0	182
San Marcos*	199,017	376	30.0	80
Totonicapán	99,819	163	21.7	134
Zacapa	34,398	232	8.3	36

(--*Departments with predominantly *Indio* populations)

Source: U.S. Department of State, "Documents Relating to the Internal Affairs of Guatemala, 1910-29, microfilm, roll #20; *Archivo General de Centro América, Memoria*-1919, 20, and *Gobernación*, legajo 28399.

Though probably broadly representative, these figures have some specific defects. For example, those for the department of Guatemala, when compared with the city, suggest, and this was probably generally the case, undercounting in the rural areas. Those from Chimaltenango are clearly useless; the department rarely reported its daily figures, and the governor seems to have been more than usually incompetent. The published figures for San Marcos were in error by a factor of more than ten, the result of a copying mistake. They are reconstructed here from the original manuscript, but in most cases such primary sources are not available. As a result, it is not clear to what extent wide differences between neighboring and similar areas (e.g., the departments of Escuintla and Amatitlán or San Marcos and

Retalhuleu) reflect defects in the statistics or the notoriously uneven impact of the epidemic, reported in all countries. The newspaper also accused the governors of purposely falsifying figures, either to make themselves look good or to guarantee a pool of uncounted workers they could later supply for their own profit to the coffee growers as *mandamiento* (corvee or forced wage labor).[60] Nevertheless, the differential mortality of the "*indio*" departments is clear and would certainly be more so were it not for underreporting of deaths.

Table 9.6

Mortality and Birth Rates of Ladino and Indio Population (per 1000)

	Mortality			*Birth Rate*		
	Ladino	*Indio*	*All*	*Ladino*	*Indio*	*All*
1914	22	19	20	38	41	40
1915	28	27	28	40	38	39
1916	26	23	24	36	36	36
1917	25	26	26	35	41	39
1918	27	36	33	39	38	38
1919	31	33	32	36	33	34
1920	20	18	19	43	42	42
1921	21	16	17	43	41	42
1922	22	18	19	45	41	43

Source: *Ministerio de Fomento, Memoria*-1923 (Guatemala, 1923), 348.

Here the differential impact of the influenza on the *indio* population is again evident, and, again, it would certainly be even more so were it possible to correct for deaths not counted. Because *indios* tended to live dispersed in rural areas and to register their children later than did the urban-dwelling *ladinos*, babies which died in the first days or weeks commonly went unreported and did not appear in the statistics. Underreporting shows up in normal years in the very unlikely lower mortality rate for *indios* than *ladinos* shown in published statistics. Influenza clearly hit the *indios* massively, raising their reported mortality rate above that of the *ladinos* for almost the only years in this period. Birth rate figures indicate a

[60]This was based on the 5,904 treated by the *canton* doctors plus 1,476 "well off" who went to their own doctors and surely is an underestimate. Many of the poor saw no doctor.

higher than normal level of infant mortality in the influenza years; again, full statistics would undoubtedly have driven this up further. Observers reported that among the *indios* the epidemic hit women, and as a result, young children, particularly hard.[61]

Table 9.7

Mortality by Age (per 1000)

	1-10	*20-30*	*30-40*	*All*
1914	32.72	13.45	15.00	20.48
1915	46.02	16.68	18.09	27.31
1916	36.60	16.86	17.88	23.97
1917	40.59	17.97	19.31	25.88
1918	45.31	28.94	30.18	33.04
1919	42.14	33.30	29.25	32.34
1920	30.38	12.93	14.26	18.69
1921	29.11	12.39	12.34	17.86
1922	35.11	12.20	12.24	19.24

Source: *Ministerio de Fomento, Memoria-1924* (Guatemala, 1924), anexo #10.

Whereas the combined death rate for the years 1918-19 rose some 50% over the average for 1914-17 and 1920-22[62] and that of children climbed by 27%, for individuals 20-40 it doubled! This is an indication of the famous "W" mortality curve noted in most countries attacked by the 1918-19 influenza. The governor of Quezaltenango observed that "the most alarming aspect of the present epidemic is its impact on men 18-40 years old." Of the better-off classes, he said, relatively few of the young or old died but rather a disproportionate number of healthy young men.[63] In fact, among the poor, many of whom already suffered chronic health and nutrition problems, influenza no doubt killed young men, but it also carried off the weakest, e.g.,

---

[61] *Diario de Centro América*, Mar. 6, 1919.

[62] *Ibid.*, Feb. 4, 1919.

[63] For an example of the *indios* problems under the assault of the epidemic see *Ibid.*, Jan. 13, 1919.

the old and the very young, in large numbers, as did all influenza epidemics. The disease made a clean and largely indiscriminate sweep. Among the healthier elements of Guatemalan society, on the other hand, it showed the more selective pattern apparent in wealthier countries.

What were the results for Guatemala of the great influenza pandemic of 1918-19? Perhaps surprisingly, they seem to have been extremely limited. The published figures claim that some 50,000,[64] or 3% of the population, died; certainly the real figure was at least twice that, and it may have been much more. There is no way to tell. But the blow was short and sharp and the population seems to have recovered quickly. Planters and the newspaper worried about lost production and the possibility of a shortage of workers, but export statistics indicate no significant problems developed for coffee:

Table 9.8

Coffee Exports by Year
(In quintales--units of 100 pounds)

1914	831,341 qq.	1918	782,520 qq.
1915	775,631 qq.	1919	896,670 qq.
1916	874,696 qq.	1920	939,539 qq.
1917	908,878 qq.	1921	935,261 qq.

Source: Chester L. Jones, *Guatemala, Past and Present* (New York, 1966), 210.

The lack of an evident impact helped convince the planters that they no longer had need of the old system of forced labor; in 1920 the government ended *mandamientos*.[65] The influenza epidemic was yet another blow to the already greatly deteriorated economic and social situation of Guatemala's *indios* and the *indio* communities, but the absolute size of the indigenous population in Guatemala grew rapidly in succeeding years, and they quickly made up the lost numbers.

---

[64]The very low figures for the years 1920-22 are almost certainly an artifice of a new regime intent on showing how things had improved after the overthrow of the Estrada Cabrera dictatorship in 1920.

[65]*Ibid.*, Jan 16, 1919.

The epidemic did provide an opportunity for dissatisfied elements to step up their attack on Estrada Cabrera's archaic and bankrupt state. Open criticism of the President was still out of the question, but writers in the *Diario de Centro América* savaged his subordinates. Officials in the capital had no idea what was going on in the countryside and on the *fincas*.[66] The *indios* of San Cristobal Totonicapán were dying in huge numbers, and the governor and town council did nothing.[67] People could not bury the dead because the judges who were supposed to provide death certificates had fled.[68] Local authorities remained so backward, a correspondent complained, that, at the height of the epidemic, they allowed religious pilgrims to travel to the shrine at Esquipulas.[69] The governor of Mazatenango was "indifferent" to the epidemic and that of Quiché "known for his negligence."[70] In other areas, the authorities "turned their back"[71] on the problems caused by the epidemic or sought to turn it to their own profit, charging heavy fines for real or imagined infractions of the sanitation regulations.[72] Together with the earthquakes of 1917-18, the influenza epidemic probably had its greatest impact at the political level, revealing the extent of decay in the Estrada Cabrera regime and spurring active

---

[66]The published figure was 43,733: Gobernación, *Memoria-1919*, 20. But, just correcting the copying error for San Marcos raises this to 48,602, and many of the other departments' figures surely underestimated the number who died.

[67]On changes in the labor systems, see David McCreery, "Wage Labor, Free Labor, and Vagrancy Lawt: The Transition to Capitalism in Guatemala, 1920-1945," in William Roseberry (ed.), *Coffee, Social Class, and Change in Latin America* [tentative title] (Baltimore, forthcoming).

[68]*Diario de Centro América*, Jan. 14, 1919.

[69]*Ibid.*, Jan. 17, 1919.

[70]A.G.C.A., Gobernación, legajo 29399.

[71]*Diario de Centro América*, Jan. 4, 1919. In fact, the paper reported three days later that the travelers had been turned back.

[72]*Ibid.*, Jan. 10, 1919.

opposition: "by 1919 *sub rosa* opposition to the dictator had become widespread, and before the year was well advanced had begun to crystallize."[73]

[73]*Ibid.*, Jan. 11, 1919.

Chapter 10: Rio de Janeiro

Sam Adamo

This chapter examines the effect of the devastating fall wave upon the city of Rio de Janeiro, Brazil. As in most major urban centers throughout the world, the virus caused massive social and economic disruptions in Rio that temporarily halted everyday life. Available documentation suggests the disease had more pronounced and severe effects in cities like Rio than it had in the developed world's major urban centers. Although most of the city's residents were unprepared for the virus's onslaught, the poor and indigent, among whom blacks were overrepresented, faced almost insurmountable odds in defending themselves and their families.

Rio's nonwhite population had been freed from slavery for only thirty years. They occupied the bottom rungs of society's socioeconomic ladder with little hope for upward mobility. Massive foreign immigration prevented most upward mobility for blacks until the end of World War II. They worked in the lowest paying jobs, they were subject to severe under and unemployment, they lived in the worst housing, they had the poorest diets, and they had the highest mortality rate of all the city's various racial and ethnic groups. It is no wonder that the disease caused severe mortality among the city's blacks and mulattoes. This chapter will not only trace the city's mortality trends during the fatal fall wave, but also highlight the breakdown of the city's social and economic institutions and the effect upon the city's poor.

At first 1918 seemed to hold great promise for most of the city's citizenry. Most residents interpreted the string of convincing Allied victories as a prelude to peace and renewed prosperity. The daily accounts of the war's progress, along with wartime censorship obscured, at first, the ominous and ever-increasing number of deaths from influenza. Until the pandemic's fateful fall outbreak, influenza had largely been ignored as a major cause of death, not only in Rio, but throughout the world.[1] People who had read daily of the war's terrible toll in men and materiel were about to heave a collective sigh of relief as the hostilities began to wind down. Little did they realize that nature was about to unleash a cruel form of biological warfare which in a few short months would kill more people than the war.

Rio had fought a long, arduous battle against the many and varied epidemic and contagious diseases endemic to the city. The eradication of yellow fever, typhoid, diphtheria, measles, and malaria in the late nineteenth and early twentieth centuries was an important victory in Rio's public health campaign. The presence of so many deadly diseases made it easy to overlook something which had, heretofore, been an inconspicuous killer.[2] The mild spring wave of influenza which spread through the United States provided no warning of the virus's deadly mutation which would kill millions later in the year. Rio's public officials, health care professionals and the public all but ignored the disease until it was upon them. News from the front dominated every daily newspaper's coverage. Wartime censorship made information about the disease difficult to compile. The belligerent nations did not want one another to know the extent of the virus's devastation of their respective

---

[1]Charles H. Stewart Harris, Geoffrey C. Schild, and John S. Oxford, *Influenza: The Virus and the Disease* (London, 1985), 118.

[2]Sam Adamo, "The Broken Promise: Race, Health and Justice in Rio de Janeiro, 1890-1940," (Ph.D. Diss. University of New Mexico, 1983), 121-42. For additional details and information on Rio de Janeiro's public health campaign see Donald B. Cooper, "Brazil's Long Fight Against Epidemic Disease, with a Special Emphasis on Yellow Fever," *New York Academy of Medicine*, 51 (1977): 672-96.

armies.[3] The influenza epidemic's association with Spain was largely a consequence of that nation's neutrality. Spain's uncensored news coverage resulted in the erroneous "Spanish Influenza" label.[4]

By September's closing days, however, Rio was receiving daily reports of the disease's rampage through Spain and Portugal. The "alarming news" from Europe indicated that the virus was "harvesting" lives throughout the continent.[5] Despite Europe's news of gloom and doom, venerable Brazilian physicians like Dr. Olympico Fonseca, the secretary general of Brazil's Academy of Medicine, boasted that Brazilians were familiar with the "grippe" (influenza), and it did not carry anything for them to fear.[6]

Contemporary accounts indicate the first documented cases of influenza arrived in Brazil aboard the *Demarara*. The illness erupted during the ship's crossing from Europe, running rampant through crew and passengers alike. A second class passenger indicated that more than twenty bodies were tossed overboard in one day. The condition of the vessel's passengers and crew received a great deal of attention from both the public health authorities and the press. Rio officials reassured the public that appropriate preventive measures were taken to insure both passenger and public safety. Despite the precautions, one newspaper ominously reported that an unidentified woman managed to debark with her gravely ill daughter, thus eluding quarantine measures.[7] Public health authorities spent the next few days reassuring the public ". . . that not one case of Spanish Influenza arrived" in the city. All incoming vessels were disinfected and the sick were hospitalized until they recovered. The quarantine measures enacted by the

---

[3]Alfred Crosby, *Epidemic and Peace, 1918* (Westport, CT, 1976), 26. Field Marshall Erich von Ludendorf indicated that Germany's July, 1918, offensive, which almost won the war, failed as a consequence of the virus's spread among his troops.

[4]Gerald F. Pyle, *The Diffusion of Influenza Patterns and Paradigms* (Totowa, N.J., 1984), 40-41.

[5]*Correio da Manhã*, Sept. 22, 1918.

[6]*Ibid.*, Sept. 28, 1918.

[7]*Ibid.*, Sept. 25, 1918.

local authorities in the closing days of September appeared to be successful. News of the malady almost disappeared from journals whose occasional articles discussed scientific theories about the disease or its effects upon Europe. Most residents of Rio probably believed they had avoided the illness which was preying upon the rest of the world. Less than two weeks later, life in Brazil's largest, most modern city would be turned completely inside out.[8]

In order to fully understand the disease's catastrophic proportions and its effects upon Rio, one must carefully examine mortality rates. Prior to October, 1918, influenza was an inconspicuous and inconsequential cause of death. Diseases like tuberculosis and gastroenteritis were well-known disorders with symptoms and effects which were widely understood by Rio's diverse ethnic and racial groups. Rio was a rapidly growing urban center that only recently shed its nineteenth century image of a tropical hell-hole. Continuous public health and education campaigns had substantially lowered mortality rates throughout the city, but Rio's poor and disadvantaged exhibited mortality rates disproportionate to their numbers in the population at large.

By 1920, foreigners comprised almost 21% of the city's total population and over 30% of its white population. Rio's immigrants, like most foreign born of the era, worked in low paying manual, semi-skilled and skilled occupations. Despite the arduous lives the newcomers led, they were, as a group, socially, economically, and politically superior to Rio's nonwhite population, which comprised approximately 32% of the city's total population in 1920. Although racial differentials are apparent in the following analysis, nonwhite births and deaths were always underreported until the 1930s, consequently the published data underestimate black and mulatto mortality during the pandemic. The community's vital statistics collection improved substantially by 1940 and the data show nonwhite mortality was almost 42% greater than that of whites. The latter statistical

---

[8] *Ibid.*, Sept. 27, 28, 29, 30, Oct. 9, 1918.

differential offers some insight into mortality of Rio's nonwhite community a generation earlier.[9]

Monthly statistics illustrate not only the influenza's surprisingly sudden onset, but also its equally rapid departure. Prior to October, 1918, influenza mortality rates for the city never surpassed one death per thousand for any of the city's racial groups. Death rates for whites and nonwhites rose astronomically in October from nothing to 89.2 and 102.2 respectively.[10] Nonwhite mortality was almost 13% higher than white. Nor was the first epidemic's first month's mortality evenly distributed by sex. Indices for white and nonwhite men were 8.5% and 6.5% higher, respectively, than those recorded for females.

November's statistics showed dramatic declines for all the city's racial and sexual groups. White mortality declined from 89.2 to 32.4 per 1000, a 64% fall. Although it made a significant drop, Rio's nonwhite mortality decline failed to equal that of the city's whites. Death rates dropped 56% from 102.1 to 44.6 per thousand. Sexual differentials evident in the previous month's statistics reversed as women died at slightly higher rates than males. It is clear that by December, influenza had largely spent itself, with white and nonwhite disease-specific mortality falling to 2.7 and 3.7 per thousand, respectively.

Although general mortality rates for Rio were high for all racial groups, black and mulatto death rates continued their historic trends by exceeding that of the white population. The excess mortality of Rio's nonwhite population was shared by other underprivileged groups in urban centers throughout the world. Black and immigrant neighborhoods in Philadelphia and San Francisco had much higher death rates than those evident among more affluent white areas.[11] One study concluded that "poverty itself constitutes an added environmental burden and increases the

---

[9]Details of Rio's population growth and historical mortality trends are in Adamo, chapters 1 and 3.

[10]All mortality rates were derived from the Directoria Geral de Saude, *Boletim mensal de estatística demografo-sanitária da cidade do Rio de Janeiro* (Rio de Janeiro, 1918), no. 1-12.

[11]Crosby, 70-75, 96-99.

risk of mortality.[12] The under-enumeration of vital statistics for Rio's nonwhite population was an ongoing problem that continued until the late 1930s. If the more accurate mortality differentials from 1940 are applied to the fall pandemic a generation earlier, nonwhite mortality would have to be corrected to around 125 deaths per thousand instead of the 102 calculated from published data.[13]

The startling racial differentials evident in Rio's published data obscure the high overall mortality rate, which was far greater than those calculated in developed nations like the United States. Some of the largest U.S. cities like New York, Chicago, Boston, and Philadelphia had mortality rates substantially lower than Rio. Chicago had slightly under 6,000 deaths for the month of October versus 8,700 for Rio. The former city's estimated population at the time of the epidemic was almost 2.6 million compared to Rio's one million inhabitants.[14] Not even hard hit cities like Philadelphia or Pittsburgh which had mortality rates of 7.5 and 9.2 per thousand respectively, in the last four months of the year could compare with Rio.[15] Although no morbidity rates are available for Rio, if the 200-400 per thousand calculated for Boston is applied to the former city 219,000 to 430,000 people succumbed to influenza during the virus's reign over the city.[16]

The aforementioned figures are conservative given the claims of other scientists who indicate the virus attacked 80% of the population during the acute fall wave. Rio's high influenza mortality suggests that morbidity rates for the city were relatively high at the epidemic's peak. Within five days of the virus's outbreak in Rio, contemporary accounts claimed that most large commercial houses were fortunate to have 50% of their work forces on the

---

[12]Edwin D. Kilbourne, "Epidemiology of Influenza," in *The Influenza Viruses and Influenza* (New York, 1975), 510.

[13]Adamo, 83-90.

[14]Crosby, 60-61.

[15]*Ibid.*, 211.

[16]Pyle, 50.

job.[17] The vast number of people stricken by the disease in such a short time period had enormous social, economic, and political ramifications for the "marvelous city."

Since initial cases were little remarked, public health measures were not taken until the situation was clearly a crisis. By October 11, less than two weeks after the *Demarara's* arrival, public officials and the citizenry realized they confronted a disease which they were woefully unprepared to fight. The disease's etiology was not understood, a factor which made little difference in the end because there was neither therapy nor medicines to effectively combat the virus or the deadly secondary pneumonia which frequently accompanied it.[18] Brazilian physicians believed the disease was transmitted through the air, for only favorable atmospheric conditions could possibly explain the virus' rapid dissemination.[19] Dr. Carlos Seidl erroneously diagnosed the virus and miscalculated its effects upon the city, two mistakes which soon thereafter would cost him his job as public health director. Authorities in Rio, like their contemporaries throughout the world, instituted a variety of restrictions and quarantines in a vain attempt to halt the disease's progress. Failure after failure convinced officials that halting the disease's relentless progress was nothing but "a dream."[20]

The virus responsible for the fall devastation remains unknown; however, recent seriologic evidence suggests it appeared as a new epizootic in pigs earlier in the year.[21] The new virus was set apart from all its predecessors by its uniquely virulent nature.[22] The diseases's many unknowns and its frequently fatal outcome prompted people in Rio to

[17] *Correio da Manhã*, Oct. 15, 1918.

[18] K. David Patterson and Gerald F. Pyle, "The Diffusion of Influenza in Sub-Saharan Africa during the 1918-19 Pandemic," *Social Science and Medicine*, 17 (1983): 1299.

[19] *Correio da Manhã*, Oct. 11, 1918.

[20] *Ibid.*, Oct. 15, 1918.

[21] Edwin D. Kilbourne, *Influenza* (New York, 1987), 8-9.

[22] Patterson and Pyle, 1299; E. Harold Hinman, *World Eradication of Infectious Disease* (Springfield, IL, 1968), 8.

experiment with a potpourri of remedies, regardless of their effectiveness. Newspapers frequently published prescriptions which had little or no medicinal value. One remedy published in the *Correio da Manhã* sounded like an advertisement for a local vinegar manufacturer than a prescription. The daily claimed "there is no better preventative measure against the dangerous disease which threatens us" than two to three drops of vinegar in sugar water. Vinegar produced by the Usina São Goncalo was highly recommended for its purity and cleanliness.[23] Other prophylactic measures included a daily dose of lime juice, rubbing camphor oil on the body and drinking bottles of Rubinat, a mixture of herbs and water.[24]

Despite the plethora of remedies, quinine was by far the most popular medicine sought by Rio's citizenry. Even though the medical establishment questioned its curative powers, nationally prominent doctors like Carlos Chagas were forced to conclude that there existed no better medication to recommend.[25] Conventional medical technology's failure prompted many people to seek the protection and succor of organized religion. Residents of Cachambi, a poor working class neighborhood, held a sacred procession through the streets of the small community hoping for divine intervention. Images of São Geraldo, São Luiz Gonzaga, and Nossa Senhora de Conceicao became commonplace, not only in Cachambi, but in neighborhoods throughout the city as people sought the only means of protection which might deliver them from the awful pestilence.[26]

The intensity and swiftness with which the disease struck are hard to fathom. Communal housing establishments like *cortiços* and *estalagems* and the poor slums known as *favelas* fomented the virus's rapid diffusion throughout Rio. Residents of the *corticos* and *estalagems* were tightly packed into small quarters that frequently lacked basic amenities such as running water and sewers. Residents shared the common water fountain with a varied

---

[23] *Correio da Manhã*, Sept. 27, 1918.

[24] *Ibid.*, Oct. 15, 16, 1918.

[25] *Ibid.*, Oct. 27, 1918.

[26] *Ibid.*, Oct. 17, Nov. 4, 1918.

assortment of animals that ranged from poultry and pigs to horses. The agglomeration of humans and animals in cramped quarters without proper ventilation, water, and sewerage were part of an ongoing public health problem upon which the influenza virus was able to capitalize.[27] The disease's rapid spread was directly related to the unsanitary conditions in which most of the city's working class and poor lived. The association was not lost upon the popular press, which castigated the government for its inaction. One newspaper described the horrid living conditions in Babylonia, a predominantly black *favela* where "homes" were constructed of flattened gas cans and lumber scraps. The neighborhood had long suffered from diseases of poverty like tuberculosis and gastroenteritis. Influenza made the already unsatisfactory sanitary conditions even worse.[28]

The aforementioned misery and grief typified the disease's effects on the city's poor and disadvantaged. Contemporary sources sadly affirmed the "scarcity of resources" devoted to the poor and how it produced one of the epidemic's "most horrible spectacles," that of unusually high mortality. Medical assistance was always difficult to obtain for Rio's disadvantaged and poor, but the epidemic nullified the limited basic care available to them as a consequence of the masses seeking care.[29]

The "vast contingent" of sick caused widespread social and economic disruption which further exacerbated the virus's effects upon the city. Within days of the disease's outbreak, many basic services vital to the city's smooth operation ground to a halt. Schools closed because they had no students. Trolley lines which normally carried thousands to and from work were temporarily out of service because they had neither the customers nor employees to continue. The Central, Brazil's national railway, which employed thousands in Rio alone, was fortunate to provide even sporadic freight and transport services to the public. Similarly, the city's massive port operation barely functioned.

---

[27]Adamo, 31-37.

[28]*Correio da Manhã*, Oct. 29, 1918.

[29]*Ibid.*, Oct. 27, 29, 1918.

All of the large commercial houses in Rio had, at best, 50% of their personnel working.[30] Even newspapers like the *Correio da Manhã* found themselves apologizing to customers for their inability to meet delivery schedules.[31] Manpower shortages made it difficult to maintain basic public services like water, sewer, sanitation, police and fire protection.[32] Newspapers described Rio as an "abandoned city," its streets were empty, commercial establishments had no customers and all night life ceased.[33] So tight was the virus's grip upon the city that one newspaper matter of factly reported "There is no fear. What exists is terror. . . ."[34]

By the 17th of October, Brazilian president Wenceslao Braz called a high level meeting with his interior minister, whom he charged with coordinating the city's relief efforts. The Interior Minister immediately replaced Carlos Seidl, the public health director, whom many felt was responsible for the devastation plaguing Rio.[35] The new director, Dr. Theophilo Torres, faced the almost impossible task of caring for thousands of sick people and restoring the city's basic sanitary services. Officials called upon medical and nursing school students to assist relief efforts. Still others tried to insure the supply of potable water to Rio's neighborhoods, but service was difficult to maintain due to the demands placed upon the public systems and the personnel available to operate them. Newspapers decried the water shortages during the epidemic, but little could be done to alter the situation without the workers, absent due to illness, who normally operated the municipality's public works. Streets throughout the city were strewn with garbage.[36] Municipal officials attempted to clean the streets, but employee

[30]*Ibid.*, Oct. 14, 1918.

[31]*Ibid.*, Oct. 26, 1918.

[32]*Ibid.*, Oct. 12, 14, 15, 17, 1918.

[33]*Ibid.*, Oct. 16, 1918.

[34]*Ibid.*, Oct. 15, 1918.

[35]*Ibid.*, Oct. 17, 1918.

[36]*Ibid.*, Oct. 24, 1918.

absenteeism limited their efforts to maintaining only a few of the capital's major thoroughfares. Some suggested the city might offer contracts for the vital service, but it is doubtful that a contractor could have stepped into such a large and formidable void in such a short time.[37]

Temporary closure of the capital's major supply lines, the railroad and the port, compounded the public works inability to meet metropolitan demands. Goods entered Rio either on the Central's tracks or through the port. The emasculation of the labor force by the virus meant the railroad and the port were capable of handling only a fraction of their normal freight.[38] The city's temporary inability to import critical food and medical supplies caused a panic that produced a run on existing stocks.

As early as October 17th, newspapers began reporting food shortages throughout the city despite the efforts of the Commission of Public Nutrition, a governmental body formed after World War I's outbreak to control food supplies and prices. The epidemic's sudden onset and severity took the commissioners off guard. The deprivation and the commission's limited enforcement capabilities provided local merchants the leeway to charge whatever prices they pleased for their goods. Approximately two-thirds of the fresh fruit and vegetable vendors exhausted existing stocks by October 17th. The merchants were, for the most part, unable to secure additional supplies until the city's transportation network began to function normally.[39]

Supplies of fresh meat were equally uncertain. Many butchers reduced the amount of meat customers could purchase by one-third to one-half, but it was not enough to forestall the almost inevitable shortage that developed.[40] Demand for fresh meat was so great that the municipally run Santa Cruz slaughterhouse killed 424 head of cattle in violation of the Public Nutrition Commission's orders. The commission claimed the animals were

---

[37] *Ibid.*, Oct. 27, 1918.

[38] *Ibid.*, Oct. 12, 14, 1918.

[39] *Ibid.*, Oct. 17, 1918.

[40] *Ibid.*, Oct. 24, 1918.

not healthy enough for slaughter and distribution to customers.[41] The president met with his advisors every day to discuss Rio's deteriorating situation. by October 25th, conditions in the city declined so much that President Braz took control of all naval vessels and rail cars to facilitate the transport of food to the capital. Priority foods included such staples as rice, beans, manioc flour, corn, potatoes, sugar, eggs, milk, and meat.[42]

Governmental efforts to regulate food supplies and prices were too little, too late, to effectively take command of the situation. Merchants, frequently described as "profiteers," unfairly took advantage of the citizenry's situation. Retail goods were sold under a "shameful regimen of fraud. . . by the greedy who approve of the calamity to get rich quickly."[43] Some proprietors "without the least spirit of humanity" were so greedy that they demanded to see customers' cash before initiating a transaction.[44] Many of the merchants operated with impunity, ignoring the complaints of customers. A baker in the Largo do Pedregulho sold "bad bread," and when his customers protested, he challenged them to go elsewhere to find better or cheaper bread.[45] Many merchants were able to operate freely, not because their actions were unknown to either the officials or the public, but as a consequence of the bribes paid to functionaries who allegedly enforced the official prices. A small chicken and egg merchant whose home had been raided by the commission's representative and the police asked why the body only "persecutes the small establishments and lets the monopolists go free."[46]

Nor was the abuse limited to the food service industry. Prices on all scarce goods and services rose dramatically during the epidemic. The price of medications, regardless of their curative benefits, rose in a "revolting

---

[41]*Ibid.*, Oct. 27, 1918.

[42]*Ibid.*, Oct. 25, Nov. 1, 2, 1918.

[43]*Ibid.*, Oct. 26, 1918.

[44]*Ibid.*, Oct. 15, 25, 1918.

[45]*Ibid.*, Oct. 27, 1918.

[46]*Ibid.*, Nov. 2, 1918.

manner."[47] The cost of Rubinat, a herbal remedy, rose from an average 1,400 to 8,000 cruzeiros per bottle.[48] Pharmacies throughout the city became nothing more than "thieves' dens."[49] The failure of the city's trolley and rail services also gave taxi drivers the opportunity to earn substantial sums of money from people in desperate need of transportation. Many quadrupled their rates, charging customers 20,000 cruzeiros for a fare that normally cost 5,000.[50] The abuses fostered by the epidemic had the greatest effects upon Rio's poor, who could least afford to pay the exorbitant prices being charged by merchants throughout the city.

Regardless of the abuses rampant during the epidemic, there were many signs of charity and compassion. President Braz's family exhibited exemplary behavior during the epidemic. His son, Dr. José Braz, cared for thousands of ill patients at the aid station opened alongside the presidential palace. His wife and daughters spent days distributing food and clothing to the poor throughout the capital.[51] The Banco do Crédito Popular told public employees who owed the bank money that they did not have to pay any of their October debts.[52] Similarly, Paschoal Vaz Otero, the owner of a small rental building, told his tenants that they did not have to pay the current month's rent.[53]

The Favrica de Chapeos Mangueira (Mangueira Hat Factory) opened a 40 bed aid station to serve the residents of the predominantly black *favela* which had been decimated by the virus. The factory hired a cook for both the ill in the aid station and those who were too sick to leave their shanties. Local residents delivered the food to their neighbors on the hill in donated

---

[47] *Ibid.*, Oct. 15, 1918.

[48] *Ibid.*, Oct. 16, 1918.

[49] *Ibid.*, Oct. 25, 1918.

[50] *Ibid.*, Oct. 24, 25, 27, 1918.

[51] *Ibid.*, Oct. 25, 27 1918.

[52] *Ibid.*, Oct. 30, 1918.

[53] *Ibid.*, Oct. 31, 1918.

army mess kits.[54] These and other humanitarian acts helped brighten the gloom that engulfed Rio in the dark days of October and November.

It is evident that the influenza tragedy brought out both the best and worst in Rio's citizenry, but it is hard to understand the panic that overwhelmed the city in such a short time. The city's mortality rate offers a statistical measurement of death, but it obscures the tragedy influenza brought to the capital's people. Men, women, and children were dying so fast the *Correio da Manhã* began publishing a daily body count on October 12. By November 11th, 13,525 people had died from the virus.[55] Yet even these numbers do not present an accurate portrayal of the dread engulfing the capital.

President Braz made a speech to the people on October 24th in which he said that the epidemic's worst moments were now a part of the past, therefore there was "no reason to continue the panic so well established in the population's heart."[56] Yet even as the president spoke, the newspaper indicated "putrefied cadavers" could be found in all city neighborhoods.[57] The indigent who died in the street, without family or friends, were fortunate to be covered by a simple sheet.[58] Funerary services, like most others in the city, broke down, forcing the government to conscript men and seek volunteers to help bury the dead. Prisoners from the local penitentiary, municipal workers, and stevedores were all used.[59] Carpenters from Lloyd Brasileiro, the nation's merchant marine, built coffins around the clock, yet they were unable to satisfy the city's voracious demand.[60] The newspaper

---

[54]*Ibid.*, Oct. 27, 1918.

[55]*Ibid.*, Nov. 11, 1918.

[56]*Ibid.*, Oct. 24, 1918.

[57]*Ibid.*

[58]*Ibid.*, Oct. 27, 1918.

[59]*Ibid.*, Oct. 26, 1918.

[60]*Ibid.*, Oct. 25, 1918.

sardonically reported "the police no longer hunt the living so that they can inter the dead."[61]

The cemeteries at Caju and São Francisco Xavier employed 200 to 300 men around the clock, all with one grisly mission.[62] The dead piled up so fast, however, the government was forced to take direct command of the cemeteries. The military's obvious and unenviable task was to bury, what the newspaper described as "mountains, piles of cadavers, [all] in a horrible confusion, awaiting interment.[63] Many hoped the move would help quash the many published funerary irregularities that emerged during the crisis and that it would forestall the outbreak of other deadly diseases like cholera, yellow fever, scarlet fever, and typhoid.[64]

In some respects, the epidemic which devastated Rio in 1918 was no different than that which wrecked havoc on cities and towns throughout the world. Neither the young, the old, nor the strong middle aged men and women in the prime of their lives were spared.[65] The greatest difference in the virus's effect on Rio was the sheer number of people that it killed. Influenza killed more than ten times as many people on a per capita basis in Rio than it did in the United States. The virus left so many adults dead that it orphaned hundreds of children within weeks. The situation was so bad that it prompted the government to establish a facility specifically for children who lost their parents during the epidemic.[66]

Rio's disproportionately nonwhite poor were the most unprepared to face the disease's fury. The epidemic's devastation of the city's nonwhite community showed that little had changed since the slaves were freed thirty years earlier. Capitalism, touted by nineteenth century abolitionists as the

---

[61] *Ibid.*, Oct. 26, 1918.

[62] *Ibid.*, Oct. 25, 1918.

[63] *Ibid.*

[64] *Ibid.*, Oct. 24, 26, Nov. 5, 7, 1918.

[65] *Ibid.*, Oct. 29, 31, 1918.

[66] *Ibid.*, Oct. 26, 27, 30, Nov. 3, 11, 1918.

answer to the inferior socioeconomic status of blacks and mulattoes, had failed. The group's excessive mortality rates confirm the unenviable socioeconomic position it occupied. The only solace that blacks and mulattoes had was that the disease passed through the city rapidly; had it lingered it might have jeopardized the small but tenuous gains so far made in the post abolition era.

Select Bibliography

The items in the following bibliography are intended to give both general and scholarly readers a start into the literature concerning the pandemic of 1918-1919. For the original sources, documents, etc. used in the preparation of the chapters of this volume, the notes to the chapters should be consulted. Some non-western studies are included because the revisions of the pandemic's mortality has focused in those parts of the world.

General Studies

William I. B. Beveridge, *Influenza: The Last Great Plague*, rev. ed. (New York, 1978).

F. M. Burnet and E. Clarke, *Influenza: A Survey of the Last Fifty Years in the Light of Modern Work on the Virus of Epidemic Influenza* (Melbourne, 1942).

Richard Collier, *The Plague of the Spanish Lady* (London and New York, 1974).

Selwin Collins, *Excess Deaths from Influenza and Pneumonia and from Important Chronic diseases during Epidemic Periods* (Washington, 1953).

F. G. Crookshank (ed.) *Influenza: Essays by Several Authors* (London, 1922).

Stephen S. Hall, "The Flu," *Sicence 83*, 4 (Nov., 1983): 56-64.

Sally Smith Hughes, *The Virus: A History of the Concept* (London and New York, 1977).

Edwin D. Kilbourne, *Influenza* (New York and London, 1987).

Edwin O. Jordan, *Epidemic Influenza: A Survey* (Chicago, 1927).

Vincent J. Knapp, *Disease and Its Impact on Modern European History* (Lewiston, N.Y., 1989).

Bradford Luckingham, *Epidemic in the Southwest, 1918-1919* (El Paso, 1984).

A. S. Monto, "Influenza: Quantifying Morbidity and Mortality," *American Journal of Medicine*, 82 (June 19, 1987): 20-25.

J. Mulder and J.E. Hers, *Influenza* (Groningen, 1972-73).

P. K. Olitzky, "In Investigation on Epidemic Influenza" in O.W. Caldwell and E.E. Slosson (eds.), *Science Remaking the World* (1923), 99-114.

K. David Patterson, *Pandemic Influenza, 1700-1900* (Totowa, N.J., 1986).

Gerald F. Pyle and K. David Patterson, "Influenza Diffusion in European History: Patterns and Paradigms," *Ecology of Disease*, 2 (1984): 173-84.

Gerald F. Pyle, *The Diffusion of Influenza: Patterns and Paradigms* (Totowa, N.J., 1986).

G.G. Schild, "Influenza," in *A World Geography of Human Diseases*, ed. by G. M. Howe (London, 1977).

Kingsley M. Stevens, "The Pathophysiology of Influenzal Pneumonia in 1918," *Perspectives in Biology and Medicine*, 25 (1981): 115-25.

C. H. Stuart-Harris, *Influenza and Other Virus Infections of the Respiratory Tract* (Baltimore, 1965).

W. T. Vaughan, *Influenza: An Epidemiologic Survey* (Baltimore, 1921).

M. C. Winternitz, Isabel M. Watson, and Frank P. McNamara, *The Pathology of Influenza* (Woodbridge, CT, 1990, originally published in 1920).

National and Local Studies: Western World

Marybelle Burch, "'I Don't Know Only What We Hear': The Soldiers' View of the 1918 Influenza Epidemic," *Indiana Medical History Quartely*, 9 (Dec., 1983): 23-27.

Alfred W. Crosby, *Epidemic and Peace, 1918* (Westport, CT, 1976). reissued as *The Forgotten Pandemic* (New York, 1989).

G. M. Emerson, "The 'Spanish Lady' in Alabama," *Alabama Journal of Medical Sciences*, 23 (April, 1986): 217-21.

Philip C. Ensley, "Indiana and the Influenza Pandemic of 1918," *Indiana Medical History Quaterly*, 9 (Dec., 1983): 3-22.

Jack Fincher, "America's Deadly Rendezvous with the 'Spanish Lady,' *Smithsonian*, 19 (Jan., 1989): 130-32.

Stuart Galishoff, "Newark and the Great Influenza Pandemic of 1918," *Bulletin of the History of Medicine*, 43 (May-June, 1969): 246-68.

Arseny K. Hernoff, "The Influenza Epidemic of 1918-19 in San Francisco," *Military Surgeon*, 89 (Nov., 1941): 806-10.

Martha L. Hildreth, "Contemporary Concepts of Etiology, Therapy, and Prevention in the French Influenza Epidemic of 1918-1919," *Social History of Medicine*, 4 (Aug., 1991): 277-94.

A. A. Hoehling, *The Great Epidemic* (Boston, 1961).

Richard Melzer, "A Dark and Terrible Moment: The Spanish Flu Epidemic of 1918 in New Mexico," *New Mexico Historical Review*, 57 (July, 1982): 213-36.

Pierce C. Mullen and Michael L. Nelson, "Montanans and 'the Most Peculiar Disease': The Influenza Epidemic and Public Health, 1918-1919," *Montana: The Magazine of Western History*, 37 (Spring, 1987): 50-61.

Richard E. Neustadt and Harvey Fineberg, *The Epidemic That Never Was: Policy-Making and the Swine Flu Affair* (New York, 1983).

William R. Noyes, "The Influenza Epidemic of 1918-19, A Misplaced Chapter in United States Social and Institutional History," unpublished Ph.D. dissertation, U.C.L.A., 1968.

June Osborn (ed.), *Influenza in America, 1918-1976* (New York, 1977).

Joseph E. Persico, "The Great Swine Flu Epidemic of 1918," *American Heritage*, 27 (June, 1976): 28-31, 80-86.

Eileen Pettigrew, *The Silent Enemy: Canada and the Deadly Flu of 1918* (Saskatoon, 1983).

Dorothy Ann Pettit, "A Cruel Wind: America Experiences the Pandemic of Influenza, 1918-20," unpublished Ph.D. dissertation, University of New Hampshire, 1976.

Irwin Ross, "The Great Plague of 1918," *American History Illustrated*, 1 (July, 1969), 12-17.

Francis Russell, "Journal of the Plague: the 1918 Influenza," *Yale Review*, n.s., 47 (Dec., 1957): 219-35.

Wayne L. Sanford, "The Influenza Epidemic of 1918 and Its Effect on the Military," *Indiana Medical History Quarterly*, 9 (Dec., 1983): 16-22.

W. J. Snape and E.L. Wolfe, "Influenza Epidemic: Popular Reaction in Camden 1918-1919," *New Jersey Medicine*, 84 (March, 1987): 173-76.

van Hartesveldt, Fred R., "The Government and the Flu: British Public Response to the Epidemic of 1918-1919," *Social Science Perspectives*, 1 (1986): 35-49.

Kenneth A. White, "Pittsburgh in the Great Epidemic of 1918," *Western Pennsylvania Historical Magazine*, 68 (1986): 221-42.

National and Local Studies: Non-Western World

Mary Boyd, "Coping with Samoan Resistence after the 1918 Influenza Epidemic: Colonel Tate's Problems and Perplexities," *Journal of Pacific History*, 15 (1980): 155-74.

Linda Bryder, "'Lessons' of the 1918 Influenza Epidemic in Auckland," *New Zealand Journal of History*, 16 (Oct. 1982): 97-121.

I. D. Mills, "The 1918-1919 Influenza Pandemic--The Indian Experience," *The Indian Economic and Social History Review*, 23 (Jan.-Mar., 1986): 1-40.

D. C., Ohaclihi, "The Influenza Pandemic of 1918-19 and the Spread of Cassava Cultivation on the Lower Niger: A Study of Historical Linkages," *Journal of African History*, 22 (1981): 380-91.

K. David Patterson, "The Influenza Epidemic of 1918-19 in the Gold Coast," *The Journal of African History*, 24 (1983): 485-502.

______, "The Demographic Impact of the 1918-19 Influenza Pandemic in Sub-Saharan Africa: A Preliminary Assessment" in *African Historical Demography*, vol. 2, ed. by C. Fyfe and D. McMaster (Edinburgh, 1918): 401-31.

______ and G. F. Pyle, "The Diffusion of Influenza in Sub-Saharan Africa During the 1918-1919 Pandemic," *Social Science and Medicine*, 17 (1983): 1299-1307.

Howard Philips, "The Local State and Public Health in South Africa: Bloemfontein and the Consequences of the Spanish 'Flu epidemic of 1918," *Journal of Southern African Studies*, 13 (1987): 210-33.

G.W. Rice, "Christchurch in the 1918 Influenza Epidemic, a Preliminary Study," *New Zealand Journal of History*, 13 (Oct. 1979): 109-37.